THE TRUTH ABOUT IBS AND ANXIETY

Erasing the Symptoms Effortlessly
Diane M. Vich

Diane's Wellness & Holistic Health LLC

Miami, FL, USA

Copyright © Diane Vich, 2019

All rights reserved. No part of this book may be reproduced in any form without permission in writing from the author. Reviewers may quote brief passages in reviews.

Published 2019

DISCLAIMER

No part of this publication may be reproduced or transmitted in any form or by any means, mechanical or electronic, including photocopying or recording, or by any information storage and retrieval system, or transmitted by email without permission in writing from the author.

Neither the author nor the publisher assumes any responsibility for errors, omissions, or contrary interpretations of the subject matter herein. Any perceived slight of any individual or organization is purely unintentional.

Brand and product names are trademarks or registered trademarks of their respective owners.

Cover Design: Mirielys Perez

Editing: Cory Hott

Author Photo Credit: SnapHappy Photos, LLC

To Robert, my amazing husband, lover and best friend, thank you for all your support on this journey. You were by my side through every hurdle and obstacle. I love you to pieces. And my loving family, for all the joy and happiness you bring to my life. To my handsome boys Gabriel and Lucas, thank you for helping me see that you deserved more than a mom with constant illness and pain. Your beautiful smiles and laughter pushed me forward and make me strive for greatness. I love you all more than you will ever know. Thank you all for being with me in this journey and inspiring my gratitude every day. A special thanks to my friends who used to call me "bubble girl" for giving me the push I needed to finally pop the bubble and overcome my illness. That silly nickname didn't mean much to you, but it propelled me to find a way out of my bubble of chronic illness, anxiety and digestive unrest.

TABLE OF CONTENTS

Foreword

Chapter 1: The Crappy Truth about IBS

Chapter 2: Overwhelming Life

Chapter 3: What are the steps for Success?

Chapter 4: Undo the Root – Getting to the Root with Herbs

Chapter 5: Nurture the Body – Elimination Diet and Nutrition

Chapter 6: Let go of the Past – Mindfulness, Breathing, and Journaling

Chapter 7: Let's get Physical – Energetic Stress Release and Vocals

Chapter 8: Affirm Your Success: Affirmations, Boundaries, and Perception

Chapter 9: Succeed With Hypnosis – Meditation and Self-Hypnosis

Chapter 10: Holistic Health – Energy Medicine and Yoni Health

Chapter 11: Evolve – Self-Love and Reflection

Chapter 12: Bury the Past – Support and Accountability for Success

Chapter 13: Conclusion: Become Free Flowing Machine

Acknowledgments

About the Author

Thank You

Foreword

I am pleased to write this short foreword to "The Truth About IBS and Anxiety" by Diane Vich, registered nurse and medical educator, who has the potential to become another Florence Nightingale.

This bedside guide, divided into three sections – Introduction, Framework, and Conclusion – offers a course to a reader for overcoming chronic illnesses, chronic pain, auto-immune diseases, carpel tunnel, pyriformis syndrome (frequently over-diagnosed), diabetes, *et cetera*.

This sincere account exposes the medical system where "one-disease, one-organ" specialists mindlessly mess up the health of millions of patients by their ignorance or due to corruption. Medical doctors themselves are sick. By prescribing anti-life medicines like antibiotics, anti-retrovirals, carcinogens, cocktails, steroids, statins, synthetic vitamins, and vaccines, they created over 30,000 diseases. The authorities, like the FDA, instead of looking into their iatrogenic (doctor- or drug-induced) disorders, are making petrochemical medicines mandatory.

This is a must-read book for those suffering from IBS that helps the avid reader to note how doctors became parasites or willy-nilly medical reps of
(P)Harma Mafia.

My recent tweet sums up IBS: "Irritable Bowel Syndrome is nothing but Acidity due to Bad Digestion. No Need for Drugs, Surgery, etc. Instead, go on a diet of fruit fast, fresh buttermilk/yogurt, biochemic, herbal, homeopathic remedies for one week to ten days, and you will be fine. 100% guarantee of Dr. Leo Rebello, world's senior most Holistic Healer, nominated for Medicine Nobel."

Read this book and read all-time best-seller *Medical Nemesis* by Ivan Illich. Also read *America the Poisoned*, which deals with pesticides, fungicides, and regicides. And finally, *Doctors,*

Drugs and Devils and from being a Sick American become a Healthy American.

This book will help you to rise from the ashes. From almost death to total blossoming of the lotus of your life through Yoni Yoga. Now the author, in her "Re-Birth," should devote more time to fascinating subjects like diet and nutrition, dance and music Therapy, *Ayurveda* (Science of Life), homeopathy, naturopathy, *PanchKarma*, and yoga.

Love is the greatest gift. It's time to *fly* and be *free* by reading this book in American colloquial English, including the F-words. So, I too say, "Fuck off," to deadly drugs, diseases, and con Doctors. Welcome nurses like Diane Vich.

Prof. Dr. Leo Rebello,
N.D., Ph.D., D.Sc., F.F.Hom., D.H.S.
Holistic Healing and Holistic Development Expert since 1975,
Bombay, India
24 November 2019

CHAPTER 1: THE CRAPPY TRUTH ABOUT IBS

Mommy Issues

My client Sandy had a past that haunted her. She lost her mom at a young age, but it didn't stop her from reemerging from difficult times. It left her feeling as if the loss was her fault. If only she could was a good girl, her mom would have lived longer. Negative thoughts like these haunted her since childhood. These thoughts plagued her with anxiety and digestive issues. She thought she wasn't good enough, wasn't beautiful, wasn't knowledgeable, and wasn't worthy. It all started to emerge as a little girl being scared at school and social events. She was traumatized and frozen during tests, shows and presentations. She didn't think she was good enough or smart enough to do anything. She thought she couldn't do well on tests or act on stage. Her symptoms impacted her in all situations. Her constipation, indigestion and cramping started in those early years and progressively worsened. She was a little girl who spent hours at the doctor. She always had urinary tract infections, cramps, and abdominal pain.

She grew up to be an adult with horrible digestive issues and physical pain. Her doctor just gave her a solution she was not ready for. She couldn't accept removing an organ just yet. She came to me to find her answer. She read my articles and felt hope for her symptoms. She wanted her stomach pain, constipation, diarrhea, and cramping to end.

She wanted a life free of prescriptions. She desperately wanted to stay out of the operating room. She didn't want to stay out because she lost her mom there; she wanted it because she deserved better than that and wanted to leave all her organs intact if at all possible. She told her doctor to give her a few months to try something different. He scheduled a follow up visit for four months to schedule her surgery. She thanked him and went on a search to find her answers. She desperately searched on the internet reading blogs and articles. She came across a few of mine that interested and intrigued her. She picked up the phone and called me after reading *Hypochondriac No Way!* And the rest is history. The interesting thing she found was she finally saw her symptoms improve easily and effortlessly. As she worked with me, she finally forgave herself for losing her mom and letting go of the blame she inflicted on herself. She realized it wasn't her fault.

Some surprisingly little incidences from her childhood also became clear. She finally understood why confrontation, conversation, presentations, and social events were so hard for her. She finally understood the difference between the way she wanted to feel and how she felt. She finally started to see her symptoms disappear and become more active in life. She had more energy and went out to the movies. She was not as stiff and started to walk around the neighborhood. She overcame those silly childhood worries, and her life began to change. She got her body back. She loved to ride bike outdoors, but all her symptoms kept her bike on a rack. But one day, she got on that bike and kept riding. She worked with me for a few years on her routine to get to that point. But she did it. The best part was when she went back to the doctor symptom free. He was shocked. He ran more tests just to make sure. She reduced her inflammation drastically. All her tests and labs showed improvements. She did it herself. I guided her, but the progress and success was all hers.

IBS Sucks

Irritable bowel syndrome is a digestive disorder that causes bloating, gas, cramps, and pain in the stomach and intestines. Some other symptoms might be heartburn, sore throat, belching and farting. Haha, made you laugh. That gas, bloating, and discomfort could be IBS. It basically means anything can trigger your symptoms. It can happen anytime and anywhere. Sometimes it's food-related, but not always. The biggest problem with IBS is that it is hard to diagnose and treat. It can take months of countless tests and doctor visits before you get an answer. But even with the answer, you don't find a solution that works.

Doctors order countless tests to rule out other conditions, such as Crohn's, ulcers, inflammatory bowel disease (IBD), celiac disease, et cetera. The diagnosis comes after every other disease or condition is ruled out. It basically means there is no real disease diagnosis to give other than your stomach and intestines are reacting to something. You get a vague diagnosis that is hard to treat. I remember those countless tests like they were yesterday. But every time my clients recite the list of treatments, prescriptions, and surgeries, I remember the pain. They had radiology exams, swallowing studies, lactose sensitivity, colonoscopy, barium swallow, barium enema, and many more studies.

It doesn't matter what the test is or if it's easy to perform – the fact is, it brings great frustration. The tests take time and energy just to get to the appointment. Then you have the pain or discomfort during the procedure. And you also spend days and weeks with stress and aggravation waiting for answers, solutions, and results. You anxiously wait for a hope-filled solution. Your mind takes over with anxiety and worry because you are bleeding or losing weight, hair, etcetera. There are so many test and procedures, you are overwhelmed and missing tons of work. All this searching leaves you wondering is it Crohn's, diverticulosis, IBD, or worse, cancer. Your mind gets the better of you.

You always think the worst. But either way, you know there has to be something wrong, because this isn't normal. It is not normal to have so many symptoms and prescriptions in your twenties, thirties, forties, and even fifties. Honestly, you might not even need them past your fifties. I get it. I was searching to see if I had Crohn's, like my dad, or something else, imagining the worst. Many of your tests were inconclusive but showed inflammation and irritation. You probably have inflammation and irritation in your stomach and intestines.

Over time, the inflammation continues, and symptoms worsen. Lately your symptoms are out of whack. You tried countless prescriptions and over the counter (OTC) treatments, but nothing is really working. Maybe you are like me and had a few surgeries to overcome your symptoms, but it's still not right. Nothing truly fixes the problem the way you are looking for. You want relief, but it's not happening. You want your body back. You feel like your body is slipping further and you want it to stop. The prescription, treatment, or surgery usually improves things slightly, but it's not what you want. You want them all gone. You want to be in control of your body again.

I will share a story of a few clients using fictional names throughout this book. Their stories are filled with pain, frustration, and sadness, just like you. They also had a highly frustrating medical experience. They hit rock bottom and sought a new answer. Then, they saw the light.

Hypochondriac Heck No

By now, you might have a memory of your own that stems much further back than you realize. It could be something small and seemingly insignificant, but its impact on life is evident in all areas. Let's talk about IBS and its impact on life, career, and family. My client Amanda had anxiety and hair loss, and IBS was a huge part of her life since childhood. It impacted her every day since elementary school. As she got older, it got worse. Highly stressful situations, like exams, presentations, traveling, or public events, made her symptoms uncontrollable and overwhelming.

She spent more time in the bathroom than anything else. It kept her isolated and alone because no one understood her pain. She spent tons of time and energy at doctors' offices. She spent the most time at the pain management clinic and the gastroenterologist. If you don't know what a pain clinic is, its where people go to get injections because their pain is unbearable. A gastroenterologist is the specialist you go see when you have digestive issues. She felt like she had season tickets to the specialist offices, and everyone knew her by name. They even recognized her phone number when she called. Her files were huge encyclopedias like mine were. She was embarrassed by all her health issues.

She also spent countless hours at doctors' offices and felt completely frustrated with the treatments. She had one doctor who made her feel useless, unworthy, ashamed, and misunderstood. She visited him for years. She went to see him one day with overwhelming symptoms, desperate for help. She had migraines, reflux, bloating, body aches, fatigue, numbness, and pain. She was already taking a bunch of prescriptions, and she was in her twenties. She was infuriated with him after she shared all her pain and desperately asked for help. He disregarded her completely as a human. He made her feel like there was no hope for her when told her she was a hypochondriac. She left the office feeling depressed, hopeless, and alone. She never went back to see him after that day. She wished she stood up for herself, but she was simply too sad by his response to react.

As she told me the story, she recalled feeling a knot in her throat and tears pooling in her eyes as he uttered those horrific words. She was furious and shameful all at once. He lit a fire inside her that was not going to stop. When she walked out of the office, she vowed to find a doctor who understood her and truly cared. She wasn't going to let anyone else make her feel insignificant, stupid and shameful. She was on a quest to find someone who understood her pain, worries and fears. She wanted to find a caregiver that experienced everything she lived through. She continued with tons of health issues for years. She found a kind supportive doctor but he didn't resolve her symptoms. She was thankful she had a supportive doctor to help her battle her symptoms. But the path still left her frustrated with tons of prescriptions, treatments, and surgeries.

She suffered for years with chronic neck pain, shoulder pain, hair loss, headaches, constipation, anxiety, and IBS. She was sick and tired of being sick all the time. She was tired of spending so much time in the bathroom during stressful situations. She was sick and tired of being fearful and worried all the time. She was sick and tired of all the physical pain. She was sick and tired of feeling like an old woman in a young woman's body. But her journey to finding answers was less than over. The next decision was about to make things better in one aspect and worse in another.

Her reflux got worse by the day, and nausea was always present. Her physical pain was debilitating and frustration. It took her a few years to decide conventional medicine wasn't giving her the solution she desired. She had surgery for reflux after a myriad of frustrating tests. At first, she was better but the frustrating symptoms soon returned. Finally, her reflux was improving, and she wasn't getting sinus infections and headaches. But her bloating and cramping was so much worse. She had trouble getting gas out because of the surgery. She wanted to belch and burp, but the gas had nowhere to go. She constantly looked bloated and pregnant. She was embarrassed and ashamed once again. She was in search of a solution and real answers.

She spent countless hours at doctors and specialists looking for an answer. She spent money on supplements and prescriptions that didn't resolve her symptoms. She found herself in search of a caregiver that truly understood her, but conventional medicine wasn't working. Suddenly, she began searching on Google. Most days, the searches made her more frustrated. She often felt more hopeless and ashamed. She spent months reading blogs and searching for alternative treatments. She spent hours reading and trying to find hope for a solution. Then one day, she came across my blog. She began to read my stories and she felt the pain in my stories. She saw that I had many of the same symptoms and frustration. She decided she was so overwhelmed that she had nothing to lose.

Conventional medicine left her feelings completely hopeless, so she took a leap to change her life. After our first call, she felt safe and reassured. She was thankful and grateful to find someone that understood her pain. At the time, her biggest complaint was food allergies and digestive issues. But her physical pain and immobility was impacting her social life and career. We worked on digestion first, and then her other symptoms improved in the process. Over the months we worked together, her symptoms slowly disappeared, and her self-confidence began to grow.

I patiently sat with her each time she visited to identify the root cause of her symptoms and tackle them effectively. She told me she loved talking with me, because she felt safe and knew I wasn't judging her. She was so grateful for the support and accountability. We worked together for over a year. She established her unique healthy lifestyle and continues to see me periodically for hypnosis and body work when obstacles arise. At the end of our year together, she was energized, vibrant, and alive. She was grateful her symptoms and pains disappeared.

She truly enjoyed the way she felt with her new lifestyle choices and finally felt normal. She was extremely grateful she finally understood ways to tackle flare ups. She successfully dealt with many challenges, obstacles, and symptomatic flare-ups over the year. Now, she was empowered to tackle them daily in the moment and live the life she deserved. Over the next year, we periodically worked together using hypnosis and body work to resolve issues that would arise, but it was more of a supportive routine. She advanced in various aspects of her life and the sessions kept her feeling balanced, safe, and supported within her body. She was so grateful for everything she learned, and all the shifts she saw in her life.

Take Back Control

You can succeed and take back control over your symptoms, illness, and disease. You deserve to feel better. You want your life back, and you can get it back. You want to enjoy your best friend's party. You want to spend more time with your family and less at the doctor. You are probably too young in your mind to spend so much time in the hospital or doctor. You are in the emergency room so much they know your name. That is super embarrassing. When you work there, it's even worse. I mean, you love these people because they help you feel better. But deep inside, you feel crappy that they know you as a patient. Your specialty doctor's office always knows your name too. When you look at your file, you are embarrassed. You can't believe you were there so much that it looks like an encyclopedia. Even if it's electronic, the pattern of dates fills up your calendar.

You deeply and desperately want to stay out of the doctor. But you hit rock bottom over and over again. Your pain and symptoms constantly bring you back in, over and over again. They are so overwhelming; you make yet another appointment with hope for an answer. But the answer you want never comes. You are desperate to find an answer or solution now. You are over the constant rollercoaster. Well, guess what? You are reading exactly what you are looking for this second. That's right. This is exactly how I helped women and men just like you resolve their symptoms to achieve their unique wellness.

All of my clients have the same frustrations when they come in or schedule a call. They are all frustrated and overwhelmed. They express frustration with diagnosis, treatments, doctor visits, and surgeries. They also feel deep inside them that medicine failed them. But it hasn't – it's just not aware of this possibility yet. Conventional doctors simply don't know what you will learn with me. Because unless you have lived this pain and overcome it, you simply can't understand it.

They all tell me they love that I understand them. They

love that I lived through it and experienced pain and symptoms. Not because they wish pain upon me, but because they know that I truly know what it's like to live inside their bodies. I know what it's like to live in their shoes. All my clients love that little secret, because they haven't met anyone like me before. After the first week, they already feel changes happening. They might be small, but each of them has a smile on their faces and a pep in their step. But they all start out just like you feeling frustrated and alone.

They feel the conventional medicine is not helping them. They feel an alternative is their only option. They feel their prescriptions are only covering up their symptoms. Most of the time their prescriptions are making something else worse. They get another side effect that begins a new problem. They are sick of not truly resolving the issue or finding answer.

CHAPTER 2: OVERWHELMING LIFE

Painful Past

The absolute worst experience I had with IBS was in elementary school. I was in the middle of final exams. In other words, I was under a lot of stress that involved fear, shame, guilt and worry. I was worried that I wasn't smart or good enough. I was extremely fearful of failing. You see, I had a learning disability in my childhood. I overcame it and was mainstreamed into regular classes, but the pain still created a great amount of stress for me. I was always scared that I would get it back, like it was contagious or something. It sprouted great insecurities inside me that festered into bloating, cramping, pain, discomfort, constipation, and diarrhea.

On the day of the exams, I ran to the bathroom multiple times. Each visit to the bathroom progressively got worse and worse. I always started with constipation and ended feeling completely dehydrated with diarrhea. Each visit to the bathroom left me feeling drained and exhausted. I was hunched over crying in the back of the class. The pain was excruciating, and I couldn't concentrate. It was simply impossible to take an exam in this horrible state. I didn't tell my teacher I was in pain. I didn't want anyone to notice me. I definitely didn't want to leave because I feared failure so deeply. I worried that if I failed my brief visit back into private school would disappear.

I was worried that this test would end my emergence from special classes. I was worried they would send me back to public school. I had other fears and worries, but school was always highly stressful. That day the pain was evident in my face and posture. I couldn't hide it very long. I was hunched over my desk trying to take the test but my discomfort was visible

My teacher was calm and gentle. She rubbed my back and

calmed me down. She reassured me that I wouldn't fail. She comforted and consoled me. She assured me it was okay to ask for help and go to the doctor. I remember that she made me feel safe. I knew I wasn't going to fail if I went home. I went to Miami Children's Hospital with my mom. Countless tests and questions left me feeling ashamed and frustrated. I was sick of being poked and prodded. They asked me many questions that made me uncomfortable. I was hunched over in pain that wasn't getting any better. But the worst memory of all was the barium enema they did that day. I remember walking into this cold, huge hospital room with equipment everywhere. A fear growing deep inside me.

My brother was not allowed to stay in the room with me. My mom was too scared to go with me. I was all alone with a stranger in a cold scary room. I was placed on the cold, metal bed with a tiny hospital gown that didn't cover much. My brother was asked to leave the room and wait outside. I was laying sideways on the hospital bed with a huge tube in my butt. There was a white liquid being pumped into my butt at full speed.

As the fluid pushed into my already pain-filled belly, the pressure built to excruciating proportions. The girl that didn't speak or share her pain screamed. I screamed and cried while I jumped up from that bed. I don't know if the technician pulled the tube out or if I did. I just know that I ran screaming all the way to the bathroom leaving a trail of liquid and stool on the floor. I cried and my brother banged on the door. He was desperate to help me. I felt dizzy and lightheaded as I sat on the toilet. I felt exhausted, drained, and overwhelmed by the entire experience. My bowels were emptying from by body with a speed I had never experienced before. I'm not sure how I didn't pass out from the pain. It must have been the adrenaline that kept me going.

I finally felt semi-normal as the last drop of liquid and stool left my body. There were tons of hard, constipated stool in that toilet. I had no idea why they would put me in such a horrible predicament or why the doctor ordered such an awful test. But I did know they were not going to stick that tube up my butt again. I have no idea the diagnosis that came out of that hospital visit or the reason for the test. But I can tell you, looking back at it, that it was IBS with constipation in its early stages.

Surgery Only Made Life Worse

I was in college, and that was more stressful than high school. My gastroenterologist, Dr. Angel Veloso, sent me to a special gastroenterologist because I had difficulty swallowing and my reflux was out of control. After more tests and several different gastroenterologists, I got a solution that seemed like the answer I was looking for. My esophagus was not closing properly, and acid was constantly climbing up to my sinus cavity. It took many more painful tests to get the insurance to accept that surgery was the solution to my serious upper respiratory issues and reflux.

My reflux was so bad that I had difficulty swallowing from the erosion of acid in my stomach. They had to do a dilation of my esophagus, which means they did an endoscopy for a special procedure to help me swallow. They placed a balloon inside my esophagus to tear up the muscle and scar tissue to make the opening wider. It wasn't painful because I was sedated, but I remember having more difficulty swallowing for a few days. I was on Nexium twice a day, Reglan, Bentyl, and Zofran. These medications only helped minimally control the nausea, belching, cramping, pain, indigestion and heartburn.

The frequent infections meant more time at different doctors and more medication. I had so many specialists it was hard to keep track. The surgery was my dream solution at the time. This reflux needed to be fixed before I decided to have children. I knew that constant illness and vomiting would only get exponentially worse with pregnancy. My doctor told me that pregnancy would be horrible with my severe reflux if I didn't have surgery. Recovery from reflux surgery was painful but I was happy that I finally made a decision to change things. The procedure wrapped a portion of my stomach around my esophagus to help close the flap. They also repaired a hiatal hernia in the process.

I realized after the procedure that my reflux improved

but my IBS was worse. Thank goodness I declined a full 360-degree wrap, because I would have been even worse off. The gas during IBS flare-ups was basically trapped now. It couldn't come out my esophagus because it was closed. I chose surgery because without it, my life was miserable. It was painful and a crappy recovery, but the reflux stopped, and that was great.

I was twenty-one at the time of my surgery, and this issue continued to impact my social life, school life, and career. It kept me at doctors' offices in search of a new solution, medication, or surgery to reduce my symptoms. The search went on for years. I spent more years filled with pain, cramping, and discomfort than anyone deserves. But that seemingly perfect solution didn't solve my issue. I began to look for new solutions that was outside the box. I slowly began to remove foods from my diet that worsened the symptoms. Avoiding these foods seemed to make a difference in the frequency of IBS flare-ups. I continued on the path of prescriptions and diet restrictions for many years until I finally got fed up. After each pregnancy, my IBS symptoms would be exponentially worse, and my diet was more restricted than before. It seemed like my issues were hopeless, and I felt helpless and alone.

The frustration and overwhelm built because no real solution was available to help me with the extreme IBS and pain. I was desperate to find a real answer to my problem, but the journey continued to worsen until 2013. I suffered through it all. It continued to multiply and kept me from enjoying life until I hit rock bottom. I reached that point when my life was under huge amounts of stress from family responsibilities, work, children, and returning to school for my master's education.

A Sense of Overwhelm

The journey from rock bottom was long, torturous, and traitorous. But the beautiful gift I learned on the way is that it doesn't have to be that hard. It can be easy and effortless if you follow a unique process. My intense struggles led me to my true solution, but it took longer than I expected. I began my journey in 2013 at rock bottom. I spent six months with severe diarrhea, anxiety, chronic pain, and digestive issues. I spent all my time working, doing homework, watching my kids, or at doctors' appointments. I went through countless procedures and tests without any real answers. I was desperate to find a way out of that dark place in my life. My first goal was to stop the diarrhea. The diarrhea was constant. It took over my life. I spent more time in the bathroom getting dehydrated than anything else.

Even Nurses Fall Apart

I was a registered nurse in the pediatric emergency room. I had two little boys, who I love to pieces from the bottom of my heart. But as any parent knows, kids bring stress, too. My oldest, Gabriel, was seven, and my youngest, Lucas, was three. They were both a blessing in my life. They brought smiles and joy into my life that only a mother can understand. Dads get a little taste of that joy, but when you carry a baby inside your body for nine months, you have a unique connection. When you breastfeed them each for one year, that bond is much deeper. Stress number three: a traveling husband. He had a fabulous job but and this travel was a huge kick in the butt. I was also getting my master's degree in nursing education. Yep, I was drilling down, studying, writing, and working a full-time job. School made me develop panic attacks and my fears grew. The best part was I still chose to do it all alone. Trust me, my parents offered help. My family offered help. My friends offered help. But no way. I was an independent woman and I was going to do it all alone, even if it killed me. I kept up the charade for a long time, but my body paid for it dearly. It took a huge toll on my body, my happiness and my health.

When a Nurse hits Rock Bottom

I was having diarrhea or dumping syndrome regularly since my gallbladder removal between pregnancies. Dumping syndrome means every time you eat, you run to the bathroom with diarrhea. But this diarrhea even had my doctors baffled, and the medications were not working. He could see my hair loss and skin was getting worse too. I lived in the bathroom all the time, and my diet was getting smaller and extremely restricted. I was already on Celexa because my gastroenterologist sent me to a psychiatrist that diagnosed me with anxiety and gave me a pill. I was ready and desperate for this little pill at the time. I thought it was my answer, but the truth about all these prescriptions took me seven years to find out, so I kept covering symptoms up with prescription after prescription.

I was bloated and looked more pregnant and miserable every day. The diarrhea was constant, and I was getting dehydrated. I had to excuse myself from my patient's rooms in the ER to run to the bathroom constantly. I had to run out suddenly screaming for someone to cover me because I couldn't hold it anymore. They repeatedly sent me to the emergency room for medical attention because they could see I was really sick. One dreadful day my life as a bedside nurse ended.

My life in the pediatric emergency room was too much for my body. It still took years to find the solution, but I was on the way. The root cause of the problem took me years to figure out, but *stress* was the culprit and inflammation was the result. It eroded my esophagus, stomach, small intestine, and large intestine. The lining was all irritated, and an ulcer was days or months away. An *ulcer,* to a nurse, is not good news. An ulcer is a breakdown of the wall of your digestive tract, leaving a hole that allows the contents to leak into other parts of your body. They are extremely painful and difficult to heal. I did not want to bleed out from my digestive tract. I didn't want to die. I was scared that the end was near. I wasn't ready to leave me kids behind. I wasn't willing to leave them without my love. I loved to see those smiles. I wasn't ready to give any of that up. That meant I had to listen to Dr. Angel Veloso. I call him my guardian angel because if he didn't open my eyes, I never would have left bedside nursing. By the grace of God and the universe, my manager offered me an alternative. She saw potential when I didn't think I had any. She offered me a desk job in nursing. Finally, I was starting a new phase in my life.

The Beginning of Change

My first attempt at alternative therapy began with intense treatments, vitamin C infusions, glutathione infusions, and a *super* strict diet. The diet was the hardest part. When I tell you strict, you have no clue. It was gross and disgusting at first. It was high vegetable, high protein, no sugar, no carbs, and no fruit. Are you crying yet? Because I felt like crying the first few weeks of this. I had to stop eating everything I loved and craved. Imagine this breakfast and tell me if you could do it. My breakfast was black beans, quinoa, and salad. Yep, you read correctly. Every day, I ate this weird breakfast for months. It wasn't easy, but it did get easier as the days passed. When I wanted to give up, I remembered my adorable boys' little faces and pushed through.

I pushed through for my gorgeous boys and my amazing husband. I ate it. I took the herbs and supplements like a champ. I owned it all. I honored myself and did what I needed to do. I embraced it and I started to feel better. I did research about alternative treatments and read research studies to find a less expensive alternative for my journey. I was thankful for all these treatments, but they were taking as much time in my life as my old doctor visit routine. They were digging a big hole in my pocket too. I began to find some interesting research regarding supplements and nutrients to help with my symptoms. I researched and finally found options for my pain, digestion, and anxiety. I also began trying alternative therapies and treatments to support my healing process and reduce stress. I progressively worked towards an alternative treatment plan that worked for me. I finally had a regimen that was sustainable and achievable for my daily life.

Obstacles in the Path to Success

Fast forward to summer 2013, we went on a vacation in Mexico. I was eating that delicious, super-strict diet for months. I had a few extra options, like fruits, veggies, and fish, but the basic diet was the same. I did not eat any carbohydrates or gluten for six months. Oh boy, did I pay for it when I decided to eat it again. I ordered flour tacos; I knew corn would kill me, so I avoided it like the plague. It wouldn't literally kill me, but I knew my reflux, IBS, and symptoms would be horrible if I ate it.

After those tacos, I was back to rock bottom and felt horrible. I instantly got a migraine. It was a migraine from hell. I tried ice packs, Tylenol, and topical creams. Eventually, I had no choice but to take my prescription, which I avoided until I was desperate. I continued with headaches and symptoms for weeks. The symptoms were not constant, but they were evident and obvious. I knew that I had to stay on track and push through. I knew that I would feel better soon. Gluten was now off the menu forever. The honest truth is, I felt better without it, but it was hard to let go. I didn't enjoy having pain, feeling foggy, achy, crampy, or bloated. I chose to stay in action and push through.

More Pain than Anyone Deserves

I can tell you the journey was filled with obstacles, challenges, and turmoil. As childhood fears began to emerge over these years, the symptoms once again revealed themselves. Again, *stress* took a toll. Fears pushed me down, and I dusted myself off and kept swimming. I worked on my evolution by learning, growing, and changing. I worked on personal development. I began learning and evolving from a nurse who only focused on conventional treatments to someone that incorporated alternative modalities into her life. I kept fighting for the life I deserved. I kept fighting for the health I desired. Most of all, I kept fighting to be the mom my kids deserved. Because the honest truth is, they didn't deserve to experience a mom in pain. They didn't deserve to see me suffering. Because I lived that life, watching my mom and grandmother suffer. And that pain was hard for me to see daily as a child because I could feel it as if it was my own.

This painful story is the one that propelled me forward into an evolutionary machine. My boys were little and taking care of me. Yep, I picked them up from school with a horrible migraine, body pain, and IBS. I was exhausted, overtired, and drained. I couldn't move from all the physical pain. I couldn't get up to give them something to drink, much less get one for myself. My husband traveled and I was alone. I could have called for help, but of course, a perfectionist never does. A type-A personality that gets everything done for herself doesn't ask for help. My son Gabriel – bless his beautiful soul – he took care of me and played with his brother until I felt better. Without a mindset to change, you can't overcome hardships. Without a mindset to change, you can't feel better. That is exactly what they gave to me. My boys gave me the strength to push through. As I propelled forward in my journey, I researched and learned more about alternatives for my symptoms. I learned the intricate nature of my body. I learned exactly how to tackle my stress and felt the changes in my tissues, my mind, and my body.

The journey continued like this for years, but 2019 truly changed everything. The mind is the key to uncovering the root cause of your symptoms and pain. It all started with some evident fears that were stopping me in life and career. But without the fear of dying, I wouldn't have made it this far, so I pushed forward. Without the fear of leaving my kids behind, I wouldn't be here, so I pushed forward. Once again, I pushed forward to find the other fears that were holding me back. That lead me to a hypnosis. The fear of being seen and heard was stopping me from living the life I dreamed. These two fears were the huge part of my IBS, reflux, and symptoms. Any event or situation that stressed me out brought on symptoms. I realize now that my response to these situations was to sit quiet, hide in a corner, and avoid confrontation. My body, on the other hand, disagreed with sitting back and hiding, which resulted in symptoms erupting all over. The more upset I was, the more bloated I got. The angrier I was, the more pain I had. The more I worried, the more headaches I got. The more I hid my feelings the worse I felt. The fear of speaking my truth, giving my opinion, and standing up for myself was making itself clear. It was time for me to step up and overcome that obstacle, too. I began to learn about transformational regressions and hypnosis. It was quite a journey. I succeeded by creating a supportive routine for myself. I nurtured myself and took time to have more fun. I took time to bond with my boys and feel like a child again. I underwent hypnosis to uncover the truth of my pain and get to the root. I worked my ass off to become the woman I am today.

The routine I created took almost a year to perfect and practice. It became a technique over the months that successfully reduced my stress response. That painful path brought me to this moment to share my story and give hope to those in pain. The truth I learned in the process is that we all can blossom and emerge again. Even at rock bottom, you can evolve and grow. If you have the right support, strategies, and action plan for yourself, then the future is bright. I believe anyone can achieve wellness again. I believe that rock bottom is the first step to shifting things. I believe the pain is a sign that it is time to change. I believe the bloat is a sign that your body is asking for help. I believe the panic attacks are pushing you to evolve and change.

The moment is here. The time is yours. The only one that can decide to change is *you*. Are you ready to *thrive?* Because I can tell you the path to *thriving is resting in the palm of your hands right now*. It won't take you seven years. It won't even take you six months. Granted, some people have a lot more damage to turn around, and the process will vary. Some people have a lot more illness and disease to uncover. But if you are ready for *change*, I am here to help. The exact process I uncovered to healing, repair, and rejuvenation your body will unveil itself soon. The best part is that I did all the hard work for you. I learned, evolved, and tried a multitude of strategies and techniques. I got certifications and took a gazillion courses to create a process that works effortlessly and easily. I did it because you deserve to tackle your stress head on now.

But like all my learning experiences, the final unveiling of my process started at rock bottom. The *Unleashed Technique* finally streamlined itself September of 2019. I hit rock bottom repeatedly. It happened several times as I resisted the changes I desperately wanted for myself, my life, and my career. The gifts came when I picked up the pieces again and focused on my health and happiness. The beautiful truth is that life brings us challenges and obstacles all the time. The process I unveiled helps me dust myself off and rise again easily and effortlessly. Yep, it supports me in the perfect way my unique body needs. It addresses everything I need to push through and feel better. It stops the cramping and bloat. It keeps me calm and relaxed during stressful situations. It keeps me focused and creative in the moment. It keeps the pain and symptoms away. And it paved the way to realize my triggers and take action before rock bottom.

I created this unique plan that cuts down the turmoil and helps me fight back quickly. Now that I'm an expert at my process, it's quick and easy. You can also hit rock bottom after challenges and obstacles throw you off track. I bet if you think about it for a moment, you probably already have. I hit hard a few more times between August and September. But thankfully, I was back in motion in weeks, days, or even hours. Those struggles that used to take twenty-one days, sixty days, months, and years became effortlessly easy. That is my big hope for you. My hope is that you will find the strength to push through your pain, anxiety, and IBS. That you will get the guidance and support you need. That you will take this unique challenge for yourself. Yes, I said *begin* your transformation and evolve into the new you. Eventually, you will be so amazing at it too. It will be so easy for you to hit rock bottom one day and emerge an inspirational person the next. You can change your life. You do deserve to feel better. There is a better way. It doesn't have to be so hard, painful, and lengthy. It can be easy and effortless with the right guidance and support. Keep reading and start fighting for *yourself*. Keep fighting for your *health*. Keep fighting for *your joy*. Keep fighting for *you*. Because you deserve it. It's time for you to fly and be free.

CHAPTER 3: WHAT ARE THE STEPS FOR SUCCESS?

From Sick to Fit

My journey from illness to wellness was long and traitorous. I had months of symptoms and years of pain. I went through many bouts of flare ups, gastritis, fatigue, panic, anxiety, bloating and pain. The most important lesson I learned this last year was the mind is the key to true success. Here is a little story about overcoming obstacles on the path to success. It all began with my first appearance on TV.

This was the day I appeared on AllHealthTV for PBS. This was a stressful day for me. I was excited, but my fear was overwhelming. It was my first ever television appearance after struggling months with doing live videos on social media. It was my dream, but I jumped into it so quickly that my fears were still on high alert.

The day of my TV appearance, my stomach was a mess. I woke up and instantly became bloated for no apparent reason. I ate the same thing I always eat and looked super pregnant. The pain was so intense, I was stuck in bed with a heating pad all morning. Instead of practicing and preparing for my big day, I was focusing on relaxing. I spent the morning belching and uncomfortable. I didn't have much time to practice or prepare because I felt so awful. My symptoms were tough, but by the time I was on TV, no one noticed any bloating. The bloating, cramping, diarrhea, and pain disappeared.

I was thankful my routine and remedies worked so efficiently. I still felt a little weird in my tummy, but I was thankful no one could see it. It was more nervous butterflies than IBS at that point. My dream suddenly became a reality. The sad thing I realized that day is that my long journey didn't have to be that hard. I could have achieved my goals sooner with the right support and strategies from the start. That's when I truly recognized that ninety days was better than seven years. It took me ninety days to work up the courage to appear on TV.

It took me ninety days to learn how to decrease the bloat, cramping, and pain. Every time I fell down and hit rock bottom because my emotions got in the way, it took me ninety days to get back on track again. Every new beginning took twenty-one days or more to make the new strategy stick. It meant that each new technique would take twenty-one days to make a habit. That little detail is true for any new habit. It takes us twenty-one to thirty days to create a new habit. You have to fight your resistance to change. You push through the obstacles and challenges because we dream of a better outcome. We push through because you hope for a better life. As you begin to see improvements, it motivates you and propels you forward. You push harder and faster because you want a life free of symptoms. That is exactly what I did over and over again.

Your mind can propel you forward or hold you back. Your emotions, feelings, and beliefs impact your behaviors and actions. My naive belief in 2013 that nutrition, fitness, and supplementation was my path to wellness was only partially accurate. I thought that the solution to my problem was mostly food-related, and this little detail actually made it much more difficult to achieve my goals. I was positive IBS was only impacted by diet alone, even though the psychiatrist already put me on Celexa for anxiety. I couldn't believe my emotions were triggering those horrendous symptoms. I used the medication to hide those feelings, beliefs, and emotions that were truly triggering my symptoms. It simply patched up and covered up the underlying emotional root of my problem. That root stemmed much deeper than I possibly imagined.

The emotional root of my symptoms made success nearly impossible. My symptoms dragged on for years with only minor improvements. This little failure to recognize the importance of the emotional root made my journey take seven years. I worked through flare ups and pushed through obstacles over these seven years. I slowly made modifications and improvements to achieve success. But this last year, the transformation was much more rapid and evolving quickly. Transforming those subconscious beliefs that were holding me back propelled me forward quickly. Achievements were much easier and effective when I combined mindfulness and healthy lifestyle changes to tackle the emotional and physical root simultaneously.

This new insight helped me reduce symptoms exponentially faster. It meant my symptoms only lasted a few hours as opposed to days, weeks, or years. It meant that flare ups were no longer keeping me from going to parties or important events. It meant that my IBS wasn't keeping me from my dreams and desires anymore. This little fact was super obvious.

Now that you understand the path to success begins at the physical and emotional root, it's time to learn the *Unleashed Technique*. This unique process is the best way to tackle your IBS, anxiety, or other illnesses from all directions. There are eight crucial steps in the process, and each step builds upon the last step. It's important to have a solid foundation before you move on to the emotional release process. This is essential because it makes it so much easier on your body to truly let go of the pain. The right nutrition, supplementation, and diet gives you the energy you need to push through the emotional struggles more effectively. It's important because your body functions and needs fuel for energy, so feed it right. These are the steps in the *Unleashed Technique*.

Undo the Root

Understanding the root cause of any illness is essential. The root cause of IBS and anxiety is a combination of emotional and physical stress. Creating a foundation for yourself is essential for your journey to wellness. Addressing the physical root is the foundation of this program. This is the key to building a foundation that reduces symptoms of bloating, heartburn, anxiety, panic, stress, indigestion, pain, and cramping. The use of nutrients and herbs to reduce the physical inflammation helps tackle those pesky symptoms. Having resources to tackle symptoms during flare-ups is amazing. It paves the way to begin a routine of mindfulness to truly succeed in your goals and accomplish your dreams. Now that you understand the importance of establishing a nutrient rich foundation and addressing the root cause of the issue, it's time to take a look at nutrition.

Nurture the Body

After you understand the root cause of your symptoms, you will need to find the diet that is right for you. Nutrition is a crucial building block in a path to healing. Building a nutritious plan for you to thrive in life starts by eliminating inflammatory foods from you diet. It gives your body a chance to rest, recover, restore and repair. It doesn't take tons of time, but each person is different, and your body guides you through it. The elimination phase is a short time to identify foods that trigger symptoms and allow your digestive tract to rest. After eliminating inflammatory foods, you begin reintroducing foods into your diet. The process helps create a plan that is unique for you. It's not a diet it's a lifestyle. Using this high powered energetic fuel combined with supplementation creates a foundation for the next phase in the journey. After that your body has nutritious fuel you can begin to learn simple ways to relax and unwind to slow down your nervous system and stop that pesky stress response in its tracks.

Let Go of the Past

This is the easiest step to learn and develop. It begins with simple strategies to build a mindful foundation to tackle the emotional root. It's all about moving forward in life by overcoming triggers, challenges and obstacles. It's about reflecting on your life's challenges to make mindful decisions that will motivate you and propel you forward. You will develop unique skills to help you relax during stressful situations. Now it's time to release some negative thoughts and emotions with a fun release activity.

Energize and Release

This is the most fun and transformational step in the process. You begin to develop a routine that is fun and invigoration. Helping you reduce stress in your life by using your muscles and your vocals to address the root even more effectively. Having fun with your voice by making new sounds and singing to release more stress than you can imagine. You will be surprised at how much stress you are holding in your throat and vocal cords. It's time to let it go and free your body of stress that doesn't serve you. Releasing stress is fun and now it's time to create some healthy boundaries for your relationships to flourish.

Affirm your Success

Now that you have a strong foundation and fun routine for yourself it's time to work on creating boundaries for the relationships in your life. Affirmations are the key to success that empower you to stand up for what you deeply believe and desire in a kind and courteous way. Creating boundaries supports you in building healthy relationships that help you feel safe and supported. It's not about hurting others rather it's about making a safe environment for yourself. This process is about speaking up for yourself and creating relationships that work for you. Using positive affirmations helps you continue to build a strong foundation for your success. Using affirmations helps engrain new positive beliefs into your subconscious mind to transform those negative thoughts that hold us back. Now let's truly tackle those obstacles and challenges with a sledge hammer by using hypnosis to reframe those beliefs in your mind.

Succeed with Hypnosis

Our mind is the key to our success. Tackling the subconscious blocks from your past is the secret to staying on track in your path to success. Using meditations in your routine helps you strengthen your intuition and create a sense of balance. Hypnosis and meditation will create a sense of calm and serenity in your day. Self-hypnosis helps you create a routine that tackles those subconscious blocks and help you achieve everything you deserve and desire. The funny thing is that we are in a state of hypnosis all the time. We just don't realize it. We are in a hypnotic state when we drive to work, watch a movie or sit quietly meditating. The secrete here is to transform those words that automatically play in our minds. Creating a positive set of beliefs, affirmations and statements that propel you forward rather than throw you off track is essential. This process will open your mind to the possibilities as your new beliefs pave the way for change and transformation.

Holistic Health

You are made up of energy. Every one of us is. It flows in our bodies every day. But certain challenges and obstacles leave our tissues stagnant. Inflammation, stress and illness makes that energy get trapped inside our tissues. This step gives you easy strategies to enhance the energy flow in your body. The flow of energy helps you easily and effortlessly tackle emotional and physical stress at its core. The most fun and invigorating part of the process, is yoni health. Men can benefit from the process too. Developing a routine for your yoni (sacred sexual energy) is important for women to tackle the inflammation that builds in the pelvic to reduce menstrual symptoms, hormonal fluctuations and stress. Men also build up stress in the pelvis and will benefit from this routine. Finally you are fully emerged in your own unique process of evolution.

Evolve

Now that you know all the steps in the *Unleashed Technique* you will continue to evolve and grow. These self-loving practices keep you thriving and transforming. This is the chapter that brings everything together. It gives you easy daily routines to make the process simple and effortless. The more you use this process in your life the more you evolve into the new version of yourself you seek. You evolve and change into a stress fighting machine that tackles obstacles and challenges in the moment. This awareness and action sets you free from your debilitating symptoms. Are you ready to leave your symptoms behind you? Are you ready to live your life and thrive?

Dream

What Is Success?

Success is achieving your goal. It means you accomplished your dream. Let's face it the foundation for any successful accomplishment in life is mindset, determination and perseverance. You can't achieve anything unless you put your mind and heart into it. It's also essential you take initiative and take action. This is true for all our life achievements. It's true and evident in all aspects of your lives. You do it all the time as you progress through the stages in life. It's how you become a graduate, professional, entrepreneur, parent, investor, grandparent, etc. You learn it all along the way.

Achieving success in health is a little trickier but possible. It is possible to feel this sense of accomplishment even after deterioration and decline begins. You can overcome your pesky medical history and prove that it doesn't have to be your fate. But when it comes to illness, symptoms, and disease, there is a much more powerful hope that propels you and pushes you through it. You can feel healthy, vibrant and energetic in your 30s, 40s and beyond.

It is your hope for a better life for yourself and your family. Your hopes and desires for less pain and debilitating symptoms motivates you to push through the hard times. This hope keeps you from staying stuck at rock bottom. It is what gives you the strength to dust yourself off and move forward repeatedly. Your dream of a life where you are able to enjoy yourself without symptoms creeping up on you. You hope for more days where the bloating, anxiety, pain, symptoms, and cramps are at bay. You hope for more days where the worry and fear doesn't consume your thoughts. You hope for more energy, vitality and happiness. You hope for a brighter future for yourself. You use this hope to guide you through the obstacles and challenges. It gives you the strength to achieve your goals. You see it in many aspects of your life as you work towards accomplishing your goals.

CHAPTER 4: UNDO THE ROOT – GETTING TO THE ROOT WITH HERBS

Stressful Root

The root cause of chronic pain and digestive issues seems to be simple. Most people think it's just related to diet and genetics. That was the case with my client, Demi. She was sure that her condition was hopeless. After all, she hated fruits and vegetables. On top of it all, her medical diagnosis was following her parents' exactly. She had reflux, hypertension, chronic pain, and fatigue since she could remember. Like most people, she didn't want to hear that stress was impacting her health. You will be surprised at the transformation Demi made. But for now, let's get down and dirty with stress.

Stress and the Gut

The irritable gut is a problematic condition that impacts many people in the world. IBS is a highly complex and intricate situation to uncover and treat. The irritable gut is a digestive tract that is highly sensitive and irritated by a variety of variables. There are emotional triggers, physical triggers, food triggers, and even medication triggers. It sounds weird to think of your gut as a trigger-happy zone, but it is a highly responsive part of our bodies. Our digestive tract includes the esophagus, stomach, intestines, gallbladder, pancreas, and anus. And this area is lined with tons of nerves and neurons which is why it is called the second brain. And your gut reacts to stress with symptoms. If the two brains aren't cooperating together there is sadness in your head and chaos in your gut.

Many of these areas are highly sensitive mucous membranes that easily tear and break down when inflammation and stress bombard them. These sensitive linings are not as strong as our skin or muscles. It is much easier for stress to impact these mucous membranes and delicate parts. The interesting thing about stress is that it comes from a variety of sources and impacts us everywhere. Stress impacts our bodies at a cellular level. But for many people, the digestive tract is the part of their bodies that seems to be impacted the most. Those of us that experience IBS, Crohn's, gastritis, reflux, indigestion, or other symptoms are extra susceptible. That means it is much easier for these areas to break down, causing injury and damage to this sensitive lining. The more damage happens, the easier repeat damage occurs. The higher your emotional and physical stress levels become, the more severe issues emerge in the digestive tract. This includes ulcers, leaky gut, bleeding, tears, and even perforation through organs.

The truth of the matter is that inflammation and stress can be reduced in the body to prevent this damage from occurring. It is also possible to reverse the damage at a cellular level using nutrients and herbs. But an important factor to keep in mind is that there are two different issues with IBS. There are two different root problem areas that need to be addressed simultaneously. It took me seven years to figure out that little detail. Simultaneously working the emotional and physical root is a crucial part of the process. That is the secret to quickly impact the symptoms efficiently and effectively.

The two key factors that need to be addressed are the emotional and physical root of the digestive distress. I will cover the physical root here to set a foundation before addressing the emotional root. The physical root is usually the easiest to address with diet modifications and nutrient rich supplementation. But it is essential to remember that a truly efficient and effective transformation also addresses the emotional root. And the emotional root is usually not addressed at all thus clients are stuck feeling sick with overwhelming symptoms.

I will cover the emotional root later in another chapter. Let's get back to the physical root cause of any disease or illness. I do mean any disease process. I did plenty of research over the past fifteen years to find, understand, and impact the root cause of a multitude of diseases, including my own. The list for me was extensive with a multitude of diagnosis: fibromyalgia, EDS III (Ehlers-Danlos Syndrome Hypermobility Type), severe reflux, biliary dyskinesia, dysphagia, dumping syndrome, etc. Yep, I know I have a ton of medical issues and diagnoses. And this list is only naming a few.

The sad truth is that all illness and disease is linked to high *stress levels* in the body. Another critical factor that is building up inside our bodies from this process is toxins. Toxins are trapped inside our cells, organs, and tissues, creating even more problems inside our bodies. To truly impact your body's healing capabilities, you also need to hydrate all your cells. Our body is made up of 80% water and we need water to sustain that essential component. Fluids are important to flush the body of toxins and debris. It is important to drink enough fluids for your body weight. The fluids will also be a crucial part of a healthy functioning digestive tract. If you don't have enough fluids in your body, constipation and digestive symptoms will arise. But you will learn later in this book that fluids can get trapped in other areas of your body and impede digestive function. But for now, let's talk about stress on the body.

I was also skeptical and naïve about stress when I started the journey. I thought it was impossible to have this kind of stress in childhood, but I did. Disease and illness occur in the body as a result of oxidative stress. If you never heard of this word, don't worry. I will explain it. Oxidative stress is a form of stress that occurs at a cellular level inside our bodies. That means it impacts our cells, mitochondria, DNA, and RNA. I'm sure you remember from school that DNA and RNA make up our cells. Our cells are the building blocks for everything inside our bodies. Our muscles, tissues, ligaments, organs, and blood are all made up of cells. Our cells are constantly being attacked by free radicals on a daily basis, second by second. The thing you don't realize is that the assault occurs from the moment you are born and accumulates inside our bodies. Most infants, children, and teens have the capability of fighting this inflammatory assault because their bodies create enzymes that naturally to support healing and fight free radical damage.

The key to understand here is most children that are healthy and thriving are creating the right enzymes to address the oxidative assault on their bodies. But there are some children, like those with autism, cancer, or chronic illness, that are lacking some of these crucial enzymes. This vulnerable population would also benefit from my practice but that is a different story. After the age of twenty-one, adults no longer have the ability to create these miraculous enzymes either. The older you get, the more deficient in enzymes you become, and symptoms begin to arise. Thus, creating a breeding ground inside our bodies for assault by free radicals.

Free radicals are present in the air you breathe, the food you eat, the environment you live in, and water you drink. You intake free radicals all the time, and damage occurs every day of your life. It is a vicious and constant assault on your body. The digestive tract is the easiest part to breakdown because of its sensitive lining. The more food you eat, water you drink, and air you breathe, the more damage occurs inside you. This unique form of cellular damage caused by free radicals is called oxidative stress. The only way to combat its effects is to use nutrient rich antioxidant substances that help our bodies create those enzymes.

Some people believe that simply taking these enzymes is the best way to combat the stress. They pop enzyme pills like candy. But it is actually more efficient and effective to use nutrients that stimulate our bodies to produce the enzymes for itself. By stimulating our body to produce these dormant enzymes, you reactivate your innate ability to heal. You become superhuman healing machine. That is the secret to truly impact the oxidative stress in your cells at an astonishing rate.

The problem with supplements and nutrients is that they are not all created equal. Many supplements, OTC products, and nutrients have fillers, additives, and harmful ingredients that actually create more damage and stress in the body. It is extremely important to find nutrients that actually support the body's natural functions without creating more harm. After all, the goal is to reduce symptoms and feel better. You don't want to take a supplement that causes a new problem, which you then cover up with another supplement or prescription. After all, you are moving away from the box of conventional medicine. You don't want to get trapped in a vicious cycle once again. That would just be adding fuel to an already growing fire within our bodies. If you feed that fire, it will continue to burn until a full-blown illness or disease develops.

Remember that is where I was when I started this journey. I took countless OTC supplements and prescriptions to help me heal. But instead, I caused more damage and symptoms to occur. I knew I had a nutrient deficiency and that my nutrition was a wreck. My body was falling apart, and digestion was simply completely non-existent. I was having diarrhea, cramps, bloating, chronic pain, headaches, hair loss, and a gazillion other symptoms. I tried to use OTC supplements and nutrients that actually made my situation exponentially worse. I tell you again, not all supplements and nutrients are created equal. Not everything you see on TV, read on the internet, or find on a store shelf reduces oxidative stress.

I obviously can't tell you all the amazing supplements and nutrients out there. It would take an entire book to name them. New ones are recommended to me all the time by colleagues in the health professionals. But by now, you understand the root cause of disease and illness is *inflammation*. You know this inflammation and damage is caused by oxidative stress. The stress builds and begins to tear down the lining of our organs, tissues, muscles, ligaments, etc. This breakdown creates havoc inside your body. It damages everything, beginning with our cells, and impacts every organ. I found a multitude of products over the years that actually are truly beneficial to the body.

These are only a few of the beneficial products out there. These nutrient rich supplements and herbs promote healing and repair. Of course, "healing" is a difficult word to use because the FDA has so many restrictions on supplements. Prescriptions cause so much worse damage to our bodies, yet those are not restricted enough. I can tell you these nutrients helped me and my clients tackle the stress. They empowered the body to repair, heal and thrive by creating the optimal nutrients to fight stress. There are many extremely good products out there but finding them can be a little tricky.

Restoring the Gut

Again, supplementation is a tricky topic because of all the FDA restrictions. But the truth is, if I learned this sooner, I would have impacted the intense progression of disease and illness in my body. I wanted to learn about these nutrients sooner. But keeping with all the FDA restrictions, I will share the product names and details in a resource guide that you can access later. These are the basic facts about the products that have improved symptoms for my clients.

Nutrigenomics is the science of using herbs and nutrients to impact genetics. Genetics is your predetermined hereditary disease path. You also have genetic diseases and illness in your family history and lineage, whether you are aware of it or not. My most significant genetic condition is a really aggressive condition called EDS III. It is a debilitating condition that impacts the entire body: muscles, skin, organs, etc. It was already impacting all my body systems since childhood. The first product that truly revolutionized the performance of my cells and reduced cell damage contains five unique herbs. If this product works for someone with such a crappy medical history, imagine what it could do for you.

The question is, can you create a supportive environment for your body to thrive. Do you want to avoid those pesky genetic conditions from emerging? I'm sure your answer is yes. You can use nutrigenomics to turn off the switch and keep those genetic conditions dormant. You can even turn off the switch that was already igniting disease and illness in your life. One of my favorite phrases is, "Your medical history and family history doesn't have to be your fate." Yep, I will say that statement many times, because it is the absolute truth. I come from a family with an extensive family history: diabetes, Crohn's disease, Alzheimer's, hypertension, fibromyalgia, developmental delays, and EDS III. There are plenty more but I won't name them all. The last one is the most significant and the one that truly led me on this path to finding my wellness.

I will explain a little about EDS III, but the truth is, it is just a diagnosis. It didn't stop me from pushing forward and finding my path to health and wellness. It didn't cause me to settle for more prescriptions and surgeries. EDS III is called Ehlers-Danlos Syndrome; it is common and under-diagnosed here in the United States. It is a genetic condition that impacts every organ and system in the body. The exact details aren't important, but the fact that the geneticist told me everything I was doing was on track to support my body was empowering.

I went to get the diagnosis after a few years on my path to healing. She told me that was the best way to support my body and deal with my condition. She doesn't know the other 60% of things I figured out after she diagnosed me with EDS III, which occurred three to four years ago. After that pesky diagnosis, I was in search of a supplement that could truly impact the severe damage my body had already undergone. I was only in my thirties, but I felt like a sixty-year-old. My body was declining by the day. My friend and fellow nurse, Daisy, told me about this supplement that helped her with her multiple sclerosis. If it could help her genetic condition, I knew it could help me. That is when nutrigenomics and these five special herbs came into my life.

The herbs are turmeric, ashwagandha, milk thistle, green tea, and bacopa. But the secret is, they are combined in a perfect balance to impact the cells in exponential ways. They fight free radical damage every second of everyday. I don't know about you, but I was ready to try anything. I was desperate to find a solution that could actually heal the lining of my digestive tract. I was desperate to decrease the pain and fatigue. I was open for anything and I wanted something easy and inexpensive. You see, one of the enzymes this little yellow pill produces is glutathione. I already knew from the homeopathic doctor that I was low on it. There was no way I could afford spending another $15,000 for six months of glutathione and vitamin C infusions. I needed my body to make its own glutathione, and I needed it quick. I was thankful to find this little pill and began taking it twice a day. I was pleasantly surprised that this Nrf2 synergizer rejuvenates cells and reduces stress by 40 percent in 30 days. Nrf2 is a protein that regulates the expression of antioxidant proteins that protect the body against the inflammation and injury that occurs due to oxidative stress. It effectively destroys 1 million free radicals per second. It also detoxifies the body. It helped me produce the enzymes I was missing: superoxide dismutase (SOD), heme-oxygenase, glutathione, peroxidase, and catalase. Again, these are the same enzymes everyone stops producing after twenty-one years of age. And these are the same enzymes kids with chronic illness are missing. The best part was that my body was producing these enzymes naturally on its own.

Around the same time, I also learned that aloe was a great anti-inflammatory that was used to heal the digestive tract. But the funny fact is I am super sensitive to the taste of aloe. I am super sensitive to tastes and textures, and I couldn't drink aloe no matter how hard I tried. It just grossed me out and made me gag. I was in search of a different alternative to aloe, and I found one. It is truly an amazing product created by a physician to treat autoimmune disease.

It is a unique product made from a twentieth-generation aloe plant. This basically means this plant is not anything like the aloe plants or juice you find at the store. It is much stronger and effective in treating the inflammation which causes autoimmune disease. It has unique immune stabilizing components that work at a cellular level to create homeostasis or stability in your body. Everyone knows I needed stability in my gut. Best of all, it was in capsules, so I didn't have to taste the aloe. I started the intense protocol following the instructions precisely until my bloating, cramps, pain, and indigestion improved. It is a protocol designed to improve symptoms and promote healing. But it begins with a large amount of aloe pills that are eventually weaned down to a maintenance dose. I slowly weaned down to six pills a day, which I still take religiously to this day. If I miss a few days or forget to order a bottle, I notice changes in my digestion.

Our bodies need natural antioxidants and nutrients to support healing also. The sad truth is that you need more fruits and vegetables than you can possibly consume. It's exponentially harder if you don't like or tolerate certain fruits and vegetables. But everyone can benefit from added nutrients, including our children. This was one that I began with my kids, because their immune system was a wreck too. They were always on antibiotics and sick. They had countless infections and surgeries for ear, nose, and throat infections. I was glad that I helped them while I helped myself. The best part was that they enjoyed it so much they begged for these delicious, nutrient-rich gummies. It was their daily dessert, and they truly enjoyed it. It is still a part of their daily routine. Their immune system is rocking and amazing because of it.

These nutrient rich antioxidants change the game of health and wellness completely. You left those frequent illnesses and prescriptions in the past. You left surgeries, antibiotics, and frequent doctor visits with this nutrient rich product. This is an amazing way to get the nutrients, vitamins, and minerals from the foods you don't eat enough of. Even if you think you eat enough, your body will benefit from more antioxidant filled super healing fruits and vegetables. These antioxidants also help us fight free radical damage and oxidative stress. Some of the other benefits are improved digestion, stronger hair and nails, weight loss, better sleep, etc. My family was important to me, and this little secret gave us all back our immune systems. There is simply no way to eat as many fruits and vegetables as the ones packed into it.

Injuries and inflammation also require a little added love and attention. But people with sensitive digestive tracts usually have issues with anti-inflammatories (steroids and OTC treatments). Motrin and Aleve were taken out of my routine years ago because they continuously caused gastritis and severe digestive issues. It left me struggling to find an alternative to chronic pain, injuries, and inflammation, which is extra tricky with a condition that easily results in injuries, bursitis, tears, and pain. But thankfully, I found a super turmeric that does the trick. I found this special turmeric a few years ago. One of my girlfriend's studies turmeric and went to India to find the purest and most potent form. She created an amazing product that is a staple for many orthopedic surgeons in South Florida to help patients with post-op healing, chronic pain, and injuries. I used this secret with my clients, family, and friends. One client had diverticulitis, which is pockets of inflammation that form in the intestines when food gets trapped. She was desperate for something to help with the cramping, pain, and inflammation. The interesting thing that happened was that her knee and shoulder pain also improved in the process. She uses it in her daily regimen to help with her arthritis. But it is also beneficial as an alternative to Motrin or steroids after an injury. I use it for back injuries or flare-ups of chronic pain. It helps reduce the inflammation in a few days and doesn't cause the upset stomach and harmful effects the OTC medications do.

The last supplement I use is so special, I keep it on me at all times to tackle any digestive issues. It improves digestion and reduces symptoms when IBS flares up. It is filled with a blend of essential oils: anise, peppermint, ginger, caraway, coriander, tarragon, and fennel. These essential oil capsules create a sense of calm in my bowels that is beneficial in reducing my symptoms of bloating, indigestion, cramps, and pain. I love it so much; I carry it in my purse. I also have a bottle at work and in the kitchen cabinet. Any time my kids have a tummy ache, I give it to them too. I prefer the capsules because the essential oil tastes like licorice and it's not appetizing to me. Remember, I'm super sensitive to tastes and textures, so if that is you, go for capsules. Don't get me wrong, I used the liquid version and felt better quickly, but I prefer not to have an after taste or smell in my mouth.

There are a bunch of other amazing nutrient-rich supplements that support healing in the body. I just gave you my personal secret ingredients that helped my clients achieve success over their IBS, pain, anxiety, and digestive issues. You are free to find more nutritional supplements to aid in your journey to wellness. I urge you to lead with caution and keep an open mind to the possibility that some of them might do more damage than good. And don't worry you will have a resource guide to get all the exact details of these supplements later. It is helpful to get the opinion of a professional in alternative or functional medicine before trying new things. I am always evolving and learning the benefits of new supplements and nutrients in the journey to unique wellness. Now that you understand supplementation, it's time to understand ways to support your body in the process through nutrition.

Stress Unleashed

You remember Demi and her significant medical diagnosis? She suffered from chronic pain, fatigue, and hypertension. She was also borderline for high cholesterol. All her medical issues seemed to be exactly like her parents. She was sure that she was doomed to fail. She thought her medical history was her fate and she was doomed. But she had hope and everything changed. She changed her diet, though her cravings were a difficult battle. She began exercising and using supplementation to support her in achieving her goals. She worked on both the emotional and physic root simultaneously and her results were spectacular. Over the months we worked together, she was astonished at her results. She lost forty pounds of weight that she was trying to lose for years. Her cholesterol and blood pressure lowered, and her doctors discontinued her prescriptions. Her doctors were dumfounded by her transformation and her symptoms were almost nonexistent. Her pain and fatigue disappeared from her life. She simply couldn't believe that reducing her stress through lifestyle changes would impact her in such drastic ways. She was grateful to finally feel sexy and healthy in her body. Her favorite part was regaining her libido which she had lost years ago. Finally, orgasms were pleasurable and invigorating again even in her 50s.

CHAPTER 5: NURTURE THE BODY – ELIMINATION DIET AND NUTRITION

Nutritional Deficit

Betty was a teen with poor eating habits. She loved treats, junk food, and processed snacks. But she didn't want to keep gaining weight. Her mom brought her to me after pain, weight gain, and fatigue started to take over her life. The nutritional transformation that emerged was truly an inspiration. She also found that working on the emotional and physical root was amazing. You will learn more about her transformation soon, but first, let's learn about the fuel you eat.

Food Is Fuel

I'm sure you heard this phrase before: "You are what you eat." It used to annoy me until I realized it was true. This simple principle about the importance of nutrition began my journey into wellness seven years ago. It is still an integral part of my life. I don't think of it as a diet but rather a lifestyle. I knew since my illness began that I had a significant nutritional deficiency. It was evident in my health in an exponential number of ways. The most significant was my hair loss, which began in high school. This little torturous truth seemed insignificant to my doctors. They attributed the loss to stress and nothing else. Countless tests yielded no answers or solutions. They didn't believe I was nutrient deficient. I tried to explain that nutrition was non-existent in my life. And I knew my horrible digestion was playing a role in this too. I knew I was lacking nutrients and vitamins because my diet was less than optimal. This little traumatic symptom of hair loss progressively worsened as years passed. By the time I was in my mid-twenties, I significantly lost most of my hair, and the beautiful girl with long, thick, voluptuous hair was gone.

My diet remained poor with little nutritional significance even though I wanted to fix it. I just didn't know how to do it. I continued my health journey in search of a doctor that truly understood me. I was desperate to find someone that recognized my nutrient deficiency was a huge part of my IBS, autoimmune disease, chronic pain and hair loss. I spent my childhood and teen years eating mostly processed food and junk. I disliked vegetables and avoided them completely. I rarely ate any fruits or vegetables either, which is why I was baffled that doctors couldn't understand that my nutrition was an issue. Once I became a nurse and understood the causes of diseases and illness, I knew nutrition was an essential component. I tried to make some dietary changes, but without any real guidance, it was a hopeless struggle.

Finally, in 2013, I found a homeopathic physician who agreed with my hypothesis. Interestingly, I went to him for acupuncture but found much more. I was searching for help with my pain, but instead I found that alternative treatments, nutrition, and supplementation were essential. He was the first one to open my eyes to alternative, holistic, and functional medicine. I quickly learned the secret to reducing the huge amounts of stress and inflammation in my body. I finally started to address that underlying nutritional deficiency, I desperately wanted to solve for years.

He performed several tests, including urine, blood, and hair analysis. The results showed that I was under huge amounts of stress, which I already knew. Inflammation was impacting all my body systems – thus the multitude of symptoms, disease, and illness. He basically confirmed everything I already figured out. He warned me that if I didn't make a decision to change things now, it would only get worse. He was really worried that I was on a path to severe illness and even death.

Now, this was the second doctor who was worried I was heading down a spiral towards death. The fear of dying was prominent within me before they even mentioned it. It was, after all, my biggest fear. I was actively invested in changing things because I didn't want to die and leave my kids behind. My children didn't deserve to be left without a mom to love and raise them. They deserved to have a mom that felt healthy, vibrant, and alive. They deserved a mom that could have fun and be active with them. I knew that it all began with changing my nutrition. I began intensive treatments with him.

The most significant shift I made was diet modifications. The diet was horrible. I truly don't know how I managed to live with the super-restricted diet for almost two months. My diet consisted of vegetables, organ meats (like liver), chicken, and beans. I didn't have anything sweet or delicious to eat. I was forbidden from eating gluten, sugar, fruits, and carbohydrates. It was a difficult task, but I was determined to get better, so I stuck to it. The hardest part was adjusting to this super-strict breakfast regimen. I was used to eating oatmeal, eggs, or cereal, but all of them were taken off my diet. My breakfast consisted of quinoa, beans, and vegetables. Yep, that's right – vegetables and beans for breakfast. I felt exactly the same way. The first few days actually grossed me out. I slowly grew more comfortable with it because I noticed my chronic pain and fatigue were improving. I was thankful that it was working, but I realized it was too restrictive. Most people can't handle such a restrictive diet for a long period of time. Since I know how difficult it was for me, I created a plan than is much easier to follow. I actually progressively figured out that it wasn't really necessary to be so extreme with diet restrictions. The body can heal and repair with the right balance of nutrients and minerals by combing supplementation and nutrition. Thankfully, I help my clients in a less restrictive way. But the secret to success is removing inflammatory foods from your diet during the elimination phase. Now, it's time to understand the impact inflammatory foods have on your body.

Inflammatory Foods

There are a multitude of foods that are inflammatory and difficult to digest. These foods impact people in a variety of ways. The symptoms can include, but are not limited to, brain fog, fatigue, pain, indigestion, bloat, migraines, headaches, heart burn, and constipation. And these symptoms arise in children and adults. But there are tons of other symptoms that can arise. I began to research and identify that many of my food sensitivities fell into this inflammatory list. The most inflammatory foods – which were actually researched and published in various studies – are dairy, sugar, corn, gluten, and artificial sweeteners.

The first food I eliminated years prior to my holistic treatment was corn. I realized that corn and corn products were present in all processed foods, cereals, and baked goods. Every time I ate these foods, my fatigue, pain, and digestive issues worsened. The physical pain and digestive issues would last for days and sometimes weeks. But eliminating products with corn and its derivatives still left me with symptoms so I continued on my path to find more foods.

I still experienced the symptoms frequently, so I eliminated more foods one at a time. Gluten was the hardest to eliminate because I was a carbohydrate lover. Eating breads, pastries, cookies, and cakes was satisfying and delicious. I enjoyed every bite of these delectable treats, and I'm sure you enjoy them too. I enjoyed the smell of fresh-baked Cuban bread and pastries so much that it broke my heart to give them up. I knew that breads and gluten weren't good for me, but I really enjoyed eating them anyway. The most significant symptoms happened after our weekly pizza night. I would get bloating, indigestion, heartburn, and body aches immediately after eating. The symptoms would last for days and sometimes weeks. The worst thing for me was weight gain, bloating and headache. The weight gain really pissed me off, because those pesky five to seven pounds would stick around for days. I was bloated, achy, and fat on top of everything.

Elimination of inflammatory foods was the first step in my journey. It was a truly difficult and heartbreaking task to give up those delicious sugary treats. But I knew that my children were more important than fulfilling a craving. I knew my health was in dire need of a change, so I pushed through when cravings came. I didn't remove the gluten until I began that super gross restricted diet I told you about, which I followed for months. As the time passed, it got easier and easier to live without the foods, and the cravings disappeared. The elimination phase does not have to be as difficult or long as the phase I went through, but it is dependent on the individual and their healing process.

Sugar and Your Gut

Sugar is another highly inflammatory food that I slowly realized needed to be eliminated. The huge problem with sugar is that the more you eat, the more you crave. The more you crave, the more you eat. It impacts your body in exponential ways. By this time in my life, my digestive issues were impacting my reproductive tract and bladder. I suffered from yeast infections and urinary tract infections on a monthly basis. All the research showed that yeast loves sugar. The more sugar you eat, the more the yeast thrives and procreates. This vicious cycle creates havoc all over your body.

All my life, I loved drinking café con leche with tons of sugar. It was so sweet – it tasted like syrup. I drank it all the time and loved it. Eventually, I gave it up because of the sugar and the dairy. Now, the coffee I drink has no sugar at all. I'm completely used to it. I get the caffeine I want without the sugary side effects. It is completely different than the life I used to lead. As my body began to heal with diet modifications and sugar restrictions, symptoms improved. But vaginal and bladder infections were still prevalent. The only solution my specialists seemed to agree on was probiotics. Our immune system begins in our gut and it is our second brain. You don't have enough good flora in your system because of the way you eat. I finally realized that the yeast overgrowth in my body was caused by a sugary diet and high antibiotic use.

Before I changed my lifestyle, I lived on antibiotics almost every month. Antibiotics kill the harmful bacteria, but they also wreck the intricate balance of healthy bacteria in the reproductive and digestive tract. If you get anything from this chapter, I hope you realize the importance of probiotics to support healthy digestion. Probiotics impact your immune system, which starts in your gut, thus transforming your overall health. After all, our digestive tract is called our second brain for this reason. The gut works independently of the brain, spinal cord, and nervous system. The gut is filed with nerves and neurons making it highly sensitive to stress and inflammation. It is important for all bodily functions to have a healthy gut. If you don't support and build healthy flora, your body's natural immune functions decline. By now, you know that illness becomes more prevalent as inflammation and imbalance occurs.

Poor gut flora creates a breeding ground for infections, illness, and disease inside your body. Building my gut flora slowly began to reduce the vaginal and IBS symptoms. And surprisingly my sinus infections and allergies improved too. I began a desperate search to find the right probiotic. I tried many options until I found the right one. Then I experienced relief from the frequent feminine infections and sinus issues. I used over ten different probiotics until I found the one that truly improved my digestive and vaginal health simultaneously. There is that word again simultaneously – I love things that work synergistically to improve different issues in the body. Like all supplements, you already know they are not all created equal. But I do have a few really good probiotic options to turn to. Don't worry about the details you will get a resource guide with everything soon. Now that you understand the impact inflammatory foods have on the body, it's time to introduce a plan of action to tackle your IBS and digestive issues.

Elimination Diet

The harmful foods obviously need to be limited and eaten with caution. Now, the question is, what foods support a healthy gut? What foods should someone with IBS eat? What foods improve digestion? What foods are easy to digest? It all begins with establishing an elimination diet that reduces symptoms and inflammation. It is essential to create a steppingstone for yourself before you begin to identify foods that trigger your symptoms. It helps to establish a diet that works for you. An elimination diet removes inflammatory foods from your diet and creates a simple diet to follow for a few weeks to reduce inflammation. Each person is different, and the healing process will be unique. But this is the best way to start the process. This creates a foundation for you to reintroduce foods individually to determine if you experience any symptoms or discomfort.

What does elimination mean? It means you remove inflammatory foods from your diet to give your body a break. It means some of these foods will be eliminated completely. But some will be reintroduced when you feel better. Basically, the elimination diet is a simple diet that you will use before you re-introduce new foods. It enables you to reduce the symptoms and clean out your digestive tract. It provides your body with a clean slate. The most important thing is, you don't want to have more than one item from each food group. You stay away from most carbohydrates in the beginning, so you will notice you might only have one or two servings per day. In essence, you will have one fruit, one vegetable, one carbohydrate, and one protein per meal. This will help you identify sensitivities much easier. It's also important to keep spices and seasonings to a minimum for a bit. Try to use mostly sea salt and a mild seasoning. This is important, because seasoning and spices can add to your stomach symptoms and have a wide variety of ingredients.

Sample Day:
- Breakfast: Gluten free oatmeal with blueberries. Add a drizzle of maple syrup or honey.
- Lunch: Grilled chicken, jasmine rice, and green beans.
- Snack: Turkey slices and celery.
- Dinner: Grilled fish, quinoa, and spinach

Now that you have an idea of the simple plan, you can pick similar foods and create a meal plan for each week. Then, after eating this simple plan for a few weeks, you can introduce one new food per meal. If you experience symptoms, then you should revert back to the pre-established list for the next meal. If you experience bloating or indigestion at lunch, make sure your next meal comes from the elimination plan. You wouldn't want to add a new item when your stomach is already upset and irritated. Basically, you support your body while you feel symptomatic by eating the foods that you know didn't cause any symptoms. Then, when you feel better, you add another item. Use that item for three to four days to see if anything arises. If you feel amazing and nothing happens, then add it to your plan. If you feel symptoms, avoid it for a few weeks and try again.

What if your stomach is super upset and you have gastritis or nausea? Well, this can happen sometimes, and your body might need a little additional break to rest and repair. My secret in those intense situations is gluten-free oatmeal. I know it might not be the most delicious meal, but it aids in the healing process. I went through a few intense days in the past and actually ate oatmeal for a few days. Just prepare oatmeal with water and add a small amount of brown sugar or coconut palm sugar. Use this to replace a few meals until your stomach feels better and your appetite returns. Then, go back to the elimination plan.

Another amazing hack during food sensitivity flare-ups is activated charcoal capsules. Activated charcoal helps absorb toxins from the digestive tract and remove them from the body.

Nurses use it in the emergency for medication overdoses. But in this case, you will be removing the food and toxins that caused you irritation and upset stomach. Don't freak out – the charcoal will change the color of your stool. After all, charcoal is black. Remember, not all charcoal is created equal, so finding an organic source that doesn't have fillers or additives will help you heal faster. I also drink kombucha during flare ups. It is a probiotic drink made from fermented mushrooms. Combing it with the charcoal will help remove the toxins faster and build your gut flora. Now that you have a few hacks for times of distress, it's time to get back to your elimination and reintroduce foods.

By now, you finished your elimination diet and you introduced a variety of new foods. It's time to learn more about nutrition. Our bodies need a balance of fruits, vegetables, carbohydrates, and proteins. You truly don't need as much carbohydrates as you think. As I mentioned before, people with digestive issues actually want to avoid or limit processed foods, packaged foods, and breads.

Veggies do a body good. You need four to five servings of vegetables a day. Vegetables have the most nutritional value, yet it is the food most people avoid. It doesn't have to be so intense or stressful to add vegetables to your diet. Adding one new veggie serving a day makes it easier to make a habit. Within a week or two, that new vegetable is part of your routine and you overcame that obstacle. For example, let's say you choose spinach as your vegetable. Use the spinach in four of your meals for that week. Add spinach to your breakfast smoothie. Eat a spinach omelet for your snack. Eat spinach with your lunch and dinner. If it seems boring to you, then use more variety, but most people just need to make an effort by adding one vegetable at a time. Keeping it simple makes it easier to acquire the habit and the taste for your new veggie.

Fruits are yummy in my tummy. Most people enjoy fruits and those are easier to add to your day. You need two to four servings of fruits a day. This is usually easier because people enjoy them. You can eat fruit for breakfast, a snack, or dessert.

The nutrients in fruits are healthy for your body. Now, if this seems hard for you, then there are alternatives to adding fruits and vegetables into your routine. A great way to get more fruits and vegetables into your diet is using dehydrated fruit and vegetable supplements. They provide a nutritious balance to support the healthy lifestyle you choose.

You need lean meats like chicken, fish, turkey, and steak. But the serving size per meal should be the size of your fist. If it's bigger than that, save half of it for your lunch tomorrow. It will make it easier for you to digest if you don't over-eat the protein. Protein is the harder to digest and requires enzymes to break down. Sometimes, you don't produce enough enzymes to break down the protein you eat. If you are experiencing issues digesting protein, digestive enzymes might be beneficial in the early healing stages. But once your digestion improves, you can eventually wean them out of your routine. You can also add protein powder to your morning smoothie for a protein powered amazing breakfast or snack.

Those are the basics of nutrition and elimination. By now, you identified some foods that trigger your symptoms. You might even have allergy testing or food sensitivities your doctor already identified. You can use that to guide your elimination diet. The basic foundation is understanding the impact food has on your inflammation, symptoms, and digestion. You probably also identified some other foods that caused you symptoms based on your past experiences. Hopefully, this chapter helped you understand the importance of building a stronger digestive tract to support your immune system and intestinal function. You have a good foundation to begin an elimination diet that will unveil more trigger foods. Begin eliminating foods that cause you symptoms and create a supportive routine that works for you. I believe in you. You can achieve anything you put your mind to. It's time to take action. Now that you understand ways to impact the physical root through nutrients, it's time to tackle the hardest obstacle in the battle of IBS. It is the part that I desperately wanted to avoid, yet inadvertently found anyway. Let your fears go and find those emotional triggers.

Nutrition Unleashed

Betty, the teen with a poor diet who hated fruits and vegetables, was desperate to lose weight and feel better. She didn't want to follow the path to illness and disease like her parents. She took control of her life and ate more nutritious foods. She started a workout routine and enjoyed time outdoors. The best part was that she finally felt like a teen again. She didn't feel trapped inside her body. She wasn't stuck at home with headaches, pain and fatigue. And her new routine helped her deal with her teen hormones and unique stress experiences. She was grateful that she no longer craved high-sugar treats. She developed a gift for making paleo desserts and shared them with friends to create more awareness. Her mother was thankful that Betty's symptoms disappeared, and she was finally enjoying life.

CHAPTER 6: LET GO OF THE PAST – MINDFULNESS, BREATHING, AND JOURNALING

Emotional Turmoil

Tommy was plagued by pain and indigestion. He was in search of a resolution to his past. He knew that his emotions were holding him back in his career. He wanted to feel healthy and energetic again. He wanted to enjoy food without experiencing indigestion, cramping and pain. But when confrontations with coworkers sparked his emotions his body would go haywire. His transformation will surprise you but first it's time to understand the impact your emotions have on your health.

Emotional Rollercoaster

Our emotions play tricks on us every day of our lives. Challenges and obstacles trigger these pesky emotions every second. Sometimes, the triggers can often get the best of you and throw you off track. Our emotional triggers can create a crappy feeling inside of us that makes us want to scream, cry, or give up. The trick is becoming aware of those triggers through awareness. Awareness is a deep understanding of your body and the signs it gives you. Awareness enables you to identify emotional shifts in the moment. It enables you to recognize that a conversation with a friend upset you. Then, you can use that awareness to propel you into your transformation.

Through awareness, you can see symptoms in your body instantly. You identify challenges or triggers that make you uncomfortable. You might realize your throat got tight when your mom reprimanded you, or you got pressure in your chest after your boss gave you a new deadline. Maybe your shoulders got tense after you answered that last phone call. The signals are infinite, and your body is unique. This is truly about paying attention to yourself in different situations and understanding your unique reactions. This empowers you to use your emotions to create a plan of action that works for you. I know this is going to be weird at first, but it gets easier. The more you practice, the better you get at it.

Awareness is like riding a bicycle or learning to walk: the first few times felt crappy and you fell down often. But it got easier every time you climbed back up. Each time you jump back in and dust yourself off, the process becomes easier. Your mind, body, and soul will appreciate your hard work. Anxiety, IBS, and digestion are triggered by your emotions, feelings, and beliefs, even if you don't want to believe it. It's your body sending you messages that it is not happy or satisfied. When your shoulders get tense because your boss just gave you an unreasonable deadline to add to your busy day, you know it's a signal.

When you clench your jaw as you imagine a conversation with someone that upset you, you know it's a signal. When you get a knot in your stomach after a confrontation with your partner, it's a signal. Becoming aware of these signals is the first step. The signals can come in many different forms, which is why this is such a personal experience. Only you will truly know what is happening in your body. Only you will know that your right calf got a knot after your fight with your friend. Only you will recognize that your headache started after your friend told you something that upset you. Appreciating those little messages will begin to change the way you see your anxiety, symptoms, and pain. Awareness is the first step in transforming the way your body responds to stress.

Physical Symptoms

Your body gives you messages so you can change and transform. It sends you messages when you need to shift and move. It sends you messages when relationships aren't supporting you. It sends you messages when you agree to events or projects that aren't right for you. It sends you messages when you agree to something that is against your beliefs. It is truly amazing the power your body has to tell you exactly what you need to hear when you are trying not to pay attention. These emotions trigger anxiety, which triggers IBS and indigestion. IBS and digestive issues go far beyond diet alone. The next few chapters will reveal the true way to take control of your digestion. The rest of this book will create a foundation for you to succeed and overcome all the physical symptoms that are triggered by stress.

By now, you realized that there are emotions that trigger symptoms in our bodies. These symptoms are usually related to the emotions rather than the foods. If you are still skeptical, let me tell you a little story. I proved this to myself a few months ago. I was finally at a place where I felt calm and relaxed. I knew that my affirmations, breathing, and self-reflection had me on the right track. I saw myself respond calmly to conversations that triggered my anxiety in the past. This time, I noticed my body didn't respond. Even after a confrontation and difficult conversation, my body was calm and relaxed. I was in the mood for ice cream, and I decided to buy some. I never eat ice cream because my body usually gets gas and bloating from dairy and sugar, but I decided to treat myself anyway. I grabbed a box of Haagen-Dazs ice cream without paying much attention to the box. I didn't read the label or look at the ingredients. That is usually essential for me, because I avoid anything with corn syrup. I thought I grabbed plain vanilla with chocolate coating, which I ate a bunch of times with no issues. As I took a bite, I realized it was coffee, which used to be my favorite ice cream at family night years ago.

This delicious treat used to be a staple for all of our family night dinners years ago. But I developed a sensitivity and I stopped buying it. The interesting thing I realized now is that the reaction was the result of emotional triggers rather than the food. The bloating and symptoms occurred during family events. Of course, at the time, the food got all the blame, because that was all I could imagine. But now that I know better and saw this experience evolve, my ideas about food triggers drastically change. This time, I enjoyed the ice cream enjoying every delectable lick and bite, reminiscing how much I had missed that delicious treat. It all happened on a peaceful and fun family night without any emotional triggers. We were all relaxing in our beautiful family vacation home in Key Largo. I was calm and relaxed. I recited some affirmations and positive thoughts in my mind as I finished my delicious coffee ice cream. The affirmation was something like this: "I digest this easily and effortlessly; I am calm, peaceful, and relaxed; and this ice cream is perfectly fine for me. I will feel amazing tonight regardless of the ingredients." I stopped myself from looking at the ingredients list.

Normally, I jumped to look at the box, but I didn't that night. Instead, I drank my tea, took my essential oils for digestion, and enjoyed the rest of my night with the family. Guess what? Nothing happened. My stomach didn't bloat. I didn't get cramps. I didn't feel anxious. My tummy didn't react. During breakfast the next day, I pulled the box out of the trash to read the ingredients. Guess what I saw? "Corn syrup." Yet, nothing happened. I placed this label on the corn syrup long ago, yet nothing happened. That is because there were no emotional triggers.

I was completely calm and relaxed when I chose to eat that ice cream. I wasn't eating it to feed an emotional stress, worry, or fear. I wasn't eating it to cover my feelings. I was simply eating it because it tasted good and I felt I deserved a treat. It was interesting to see myself notice this weird phenomenon for myself. You see, I heard from other health coaches that food sensitivities are beliefs rather than true allergies, yet it took me a long time to accept that as the truth.

That night, before I bought the ice cream, I remembered my black pepper experience. That memory actually brought the truth of emotions to light. I was heading to a consultation with a plastic surgeon for my breast implants. I was going with two girlfriends, which made the situation a little more fun but scary nonetheless. I was trying to lose weight for months, but still had fifteen pounds to go. I heard horror stories about this doctor and his rudeness. I heard he tells people flat out that they are too fat during the consultation. The worry and fear about this appointment went rushing through me as the appointment approached. When I ate my chicken and sprinkled black pepper all over it, boom – I became bloated. I became so bloated that I spent the entire car ride burping and farting. Yep, I tooted all the way to that appointment. I felt crappy when I arrived at his office, but I pushed through and went in anyway. Some of the gas and bloating was gone by the time we went inside. But my stomach was puffy and bloated. It looked like a four-month pregnant belly, which made me feel even more self-conscious.

I was nervous to be naked in front of him and my friends. I was scared to show my breasts to anyone. The kids left me with breasts that were fleshy and droopy. I didn't want to show them to anyone, much less a rude doctor. But I did want to feel better about myself, so I worked up the courage and did it. I knew that my boobs looked spectacular when I was breastfeeding, and I wanted those boobs back. Truly, the appointment was not what I expected or feared at all. He was a nice old man and never made me feel uncomfortable at all. I worked myself up for nothing, because my both my friends were in the same predicament I was. He didn't tell me anything rude or offensive. He did mention my breasts would look better if I had a little tummy tuck or lost a few pounds. But it didn't sound offensive or upsetting at all. He actually was really nice about it.

After that appointment, the belief of my black pepper allergy emerged, and it stuck. It was eight years since my surgery, and I avoided pepper like the plague. Recently, I ate some foods that had a small amount of pepper without any reaction.

That is how I knew that my original plan of focusing on diet alone was *wrong*. IBS is not only about food and nutrition. IBS is an emotional response to challenges and obstacles that arise. Our feelings, emotions, and beliefs are in conflict with our true desires. Our bodies don't want to keep those negative emotions inside. The result is a message through symptoms like bloating, indigestion, and pain. I noticed over the past few weeks that my symptoms coincided with emotional triggers. When I addressed the trigger, the pain and symptoms would disappear quickly. Yep, it sounds crazy, but it would. Some symptoms took longer than others, but they would eventually vanish.

I realized that my routine of mindfulness, breathing, journaling, and self-care was working. I realized that foods were not my enemy. I realized that I did an amazing job healing myself. The sad part is, it took an extremely long time. I realized that I started backwards when I chose food as the fundamental problem. That resulted in seven years to heal IBS as opposed to months, weeks, or even days. It doesn't have to be that hard. It doesn't have to take that long. I don't want anyone else to suffer as much as I did. I don't want anyone else to suffer unnecessarily through pain, bloating, indigestion, heartburn, cramps, and symptoms. No one deserves to suffer for months or even years with inexplicable symptoms. Anxiety, pain, and IBS led to a painful and hurt filled life. It was a tough life, but it brought me to writing this book. The length of my journey doesn't bother me. I know there was a greater purpose to my pain, struggles, and obstacles. Those pesky symptoms helped me create a plan that truly transforms healing for people with chronic illness, IBS, anxiety, and digestive issues. The secret to any physical transformation is the *desire to change*. This deep desire happens when you hit rock bottom. Connecting to that pain and remembering your goal is the key element that propels you towards success. It is important to remember yourself at rock bottom while you work at your transformation. Sometimes, it's hard for us to picture or recall that person in your mind, but visual aids will help motivate you.

Painful Motivator

Keeping a picture of *yourself* at your lowest point motivates you to push through. Seeing that person in pain, turmoil, and heartache keeps you pushing forward. She keeps things in perspective and remind you of everything you could lose. She connects you with your why. For me, that was my children and the fear of leaving them alone. For you, that why may be different. But the important thing is to find a token or memento of when you decided to change. It may be a picture of that rock bottom moment. It might be you in an outfit you used to wear. Now, save this keepsake and use it as a motivator in your evolution. As you begin to change and feel more relaxed you will see the value in looking at your old self. You will begin to see new things as you look at that image over and over again. You will see the pain and struggle in your face. You will see the illness and symptoms in your body. You will see the difference it makes in your life. Your eyes will be open and ready to truly see everything that was hiding inside you. The bloated, swollen face that was hiding behind a fake smile. The woman with severe pain and inflammation that sat on a couch, unable to enjoy a party. You can use this image as a motivator and save it in various places. I saved this image of me forty pounds heavier on my phone. I also glanced at it as I passed the picture in the hallway many times. The picture doesn't trigger intense emotions anymore. It simply helps me recognize how far I came.

Positive Motivator

Maybe you prefer a positive motivator or keepsake. Maybe for you, it is better to have an achievable goal from your past. My motivator to lose weight was the opposite. Before I lost the weight, I actually used a picture from my healthier years. I used a picture of myself in a bikini before I got married to push me to lose weight. That was my goal weight picture. I wanted to look and feel like her again. Of course, in reality, she really didn't feel great, but she felt better than my thirties version. That bikini picture still hangs on the side of my fridge and reminds me of how far I came. I can tell you that I feel younger, healthier, and more vibrant now than I ever did in the past. Even at the time of that bikini picture, I was plagued with pain and digestive issues. I definitely returned to that body, but as a much healthier version.

Choose Your Potion: Painful or Positive Motivator

Now, it's time for you to decide. Do you want the positive or negative motivator? I learned, for me, the image of pain was much more powerful for me. It helped me push through the hard times. It helped me connect with my pain. It is the image that gave me infinitely better results. That image made me remember the huge obstacles I overcame. Let's get down and dirty with awareness and action. Now that you have that picture in your mind, you know the way you want to feel in stressful situations. It's time to learn exactly how to do that. How do you stay calm and relax when your friend screams at you? How do you deal with confrontational conversations? How do you blow off steam when a conversation makes you want to scream? How do you deal with sudden mood changes? How do you deal with the physical symptoms in your body?

Well, it all starts with awareness and action. You already understand awareness by now, so it's time to explain action. Action is using your awareness to release stress. Action means you make yourself the priority in the moment. Action means you step aside from a situation that makes you uncomfortable. Action means you take a break for yourself. Action means you deserve to take time to re-center and refocus yourself. There are many ways to calm the senses, relax your body, and reduce your symptoms. I will show you the various techniques in the next chapters. Now, I will focus on mindfulness, breathing, and journaling. This will create a foundation to learn, grow, and develop unique stress fighting routines.

Mindfulness on the Path to Success

Mindfulness is the first step. Your desire and decision to change began this process for you. You are already mindful and aware that your body is sending you messages. You are already aware that it's important to pay attention to the signs, symptoms, and signals. This awareness will help you address your feelings and emotions. You are cognizant of the powerful correlation between emotional triggers and anxiety, pain, and IBS. You are already attentive to the connection between your anxiety and IBS symptoms, which are triggered by your emotions. That means you are being more mindful of the choices you make.

The next step is breathing. Breathing is not exactly what you think it is. You breathe easily and effortlessly every day. It is your body's physiological response to keep you alive. But this automatic, innate breathing isn't effective in calming your mind and relaxing your nervous system. It is not effective in reducing stress. It is not effective in helping you feel calm and relaxed. But there are ways to use breathing to your advantage. That is what I am going to teach you now. There are inconspicuous ways to change your breathing during stressful situations. You can address your triggers quickly during an intense conversation. There are ways to slow your breathing to help you process and release those negative emotions. There are ways to calm your thought by simply changing your breathing patterns.

Trust me, there are many different options for breath work. These techniques were effective for me and many of my friends, clients, and colleagues in the wellness realm. This technique combines mindfulness and breathing to relax you deeply by impacting the nervous system. It begins with a simple breathing pattern that releases happy hormones throughout your body. Combining the breathing technique with the strategies in the next chapters helps to shut off the fight or flight response in your body. Let's start with the five-five-five breath.

THE TRUTH ABOUT IBS AND ANXIETY

Each of my colleagues has a slightly different breathing exercise. You can try a few and decide which one works for you. This one worked miracles for me and my clients. It will be weird at first and it takes practice to perfect. But it is simple and easy to achieve.

Take a moment to breath in for a count of five. That's right, you got this. That was super easy. Now, hold for a count of five. It's okay. Keep going. It will get easier. Now, exhale for a count of five. That is perfect. Practice the five-five-five breath a few more times, and then I will tell you the secret. Okay, so you practiced it five times, right? If you didn't, then practice it now. Ready? Okay, so now, you are going to do the five-five-five breath and exhale with an "ahh" sound. Yep, I know it sounds super weird. But it is a powerful technique. It relaxes the vocal cords and releases trapped emotions from your throat and body. Try it again. Perfect. There you go, just like that. Practice these five more times.

Awesome, you are a rock star. You just did some amazing breath work. How do you feel? Hey, if you didn't do it, then go back and try it. I can't help you if you aren't willing to get down and dirty. Go back and practice. Okay, great job. That is perfect. Now, take a moment and use your awareness. How do you feel? Do you notice any tense areas in your body? Is there something worrying you? Was there something you were pondering? Did something pop into your mind when you were breathing?

If you still feel a little stressed or worried, take a few minutes to practice more breathing. Focus on that thought in your mind. As you exhale with the "ahh" sound, imagine that negative feeling, belief, or emotion is being released with your exhale. That seems a little weird at first, but your mind is powerful. You can impact your stress by focusing on that emotion and releasing it. There you go, perfect. You felt it, thought about it, and released it. Now, it's time to dig deep and reflect. Your mind is clearer and more relaxed now. Take a few minutes to reflect on your thoughts. Take out a notebook or journal and write anything you are feeling.

Journaling is a powerful technique to release negative thoughts and emotions from your mind. You can use it several times a day just to clear your mind and move forward. I recommend journaling in the morning and any time you feel any symptoms in your body. Keeping a journal of your symptoms, pain, and feelings will help guide you in developing your unique routine. You tend to love venting and telling people your problems, but it is much more therapeutic for you to write them out and express them on paper. You can even type them on the computer. It taps into the creative outlet in your brain to release the emotions. Talking doesn't do that for us. Your only job now is to practice awareness, journaling, and breathing. The actions you are currently taking are journaling and breathing. That is easy, right? You know how to breath. You know how to write. You know your body. Get to it. Then, you will get physical as you uncover the root cause of your symptoms and pain. This is the first step towards creating any self-love routine: a decision to change. That is what will help you *thrive* with IBS. Now, it's time for you to use the journal and reflect a little deeper. Ask yourself some questions and make a list of triggers. Take out a sheet of paper and answer these questions.

- Does anyone make you angry?
- What part of the conversation makes you angry?
- Does this person trigger you often?
- Do you remember any symptoms or pain in your body the last time you spoke to them?
- Did you have IBS or panic symptoms after the conversation?
- Did you get pain in your body?
- Do you worry a lot?
- What do you worry about? Make a list. Anything that comes up for you. Then find the most important and significant thing you worry about on this list.
- How does thinking about it make you feel now?
- Do you feel any symptoms in your body?

- Think of a time in the past when you worried about the priority item on the list.
- How did you feel in that moment?
- Did you get any symptoms?
- Did you feel anxious?
- Did you have IBS or panic attacks?
- Can you recall a day that your mood shifted quickly?
- What happened?
- Who was there?
- Where were you?
- What did you feel?
- Did you have any symptoms?
- Did you feel anxious?
- Did you have any physical pain?
- Did you have IBS or panic attacks?
- Is there a situation, person, place, or thing that always makes you stressed?
- Do you notice that a certain location or event triggers you often?
- What is it?
- How does it make you feel?
- Why do you think you feel that way?
- Do you remember the last time you felt that way?
- Where were you?
- Who was there?
- What did you feel in your body?
- Did you have any symptoms?
- Did you have IBS or panic attacks?

That was amazing. You did a fabulous job reflecting. It doesn't matter what came up for you. The important thing is that you took time to think and reflect about those emotional triggers to keep moving forward. Daily reflection is easy. It doesn't have to take hours. It can simply be writing down a paragraph when something comes up. You can write it on your phone, computer, or notebook. Just embrace it and let it go.

Plan some time every day or a few times a week to continue to reflect and be mindful of your emotions. Keep a journal and use your breathing strategy to help you relax. Release those feelings with your breath. Use the journal to help you keep track of the triggers, mood changes, symptoms, and challenges that are unique for you. You are already beginning to thrive with IBS. You are on the right track. Just keep pushing through. Look at that keepsake picture. Be aware, reflect, and take action. Keep moving forward. You got this.

Emotions Unleashed

You remember Tommy? His work-life relationships were taking a toll on his health. He had indigestion, cramping, and pain. The symptoms erupted after confrontations at work and left him debilitated for days. He changed his diet and exercised regularly. He also took time to breathe and let go of emotions in the moment. He started his day with journaling and meditation. On those difficult days where confrontation happened, he took time for himself to breath and meditate. As time passed, the confrontations disappeared. People simply noticed he wasn't reacting the same and left him alone. He got a promotion to supervisor and was thankful for my support in the process.

CHAPTER 7: LET'S GET PHYSICAL – ENERGETIC STRESS RELEASE AND VOCALS

Physical Fears

Jenny was literally scared of everything. She was scared to go to the store. She was scared to take a walk. She desperately wanted to return to work, but her fears kept getting in her way. She transformed this negative pattern for herself, and it all started with awareness and action. Her energetic stress release and vocals helped her evolve and grow. Soon, you will see her transformation, but first, it's time to understand the potential of energetic release for your future.

Your New Awareness

Let's face it: IBS sucks. It sucks to feel like food is your enemy. It sucks that your emotions can trigger such an intense response in your body. But your newfound awareness of it is a unique gift, because you are aware of impact your emotions and lifestyle choices have on your body. It is a blessing to finally understand that you have the power to change your outcome. You have the strength inside you to accomplish your dreams. I know exactly what that dream is because it took me seven years to achieve it. I know you don't want it to take you seven years. You want to achieve this dream now. You want to be able to enjoy your life without debilitating symptoms. You want to live the life of your dreams without feeling bloated, crampy, and sick. You want to stop the pain, anxiety, and symptoms before they start. You want to learn exactly how to achieve that easily and effortlessly.

Well, the simple fact is that you are already on that path. You opened this book. You already read six chapters, and now it's time to take action. You already established an awareness in your life about your symptoms. Your goals are set, and your desires and dreams are in motion. You already began to establish a supportive routine for your body. You are aware of the importance of meeting your body's needs through nutrition, hydration, reflection, and breathing. Those little tasks are all creating a foundation to build upon. Now, it's time to push forward and truly release the stress that holds you back. It's time to shift and shuffle to get on the path to achieve your dream. It's time to get out of your own way and move forward. The path is easier than you think. It just takes a little practice to establish this routine. The amazing thing is, you will have fun doing it.

This chapter is all about simple little activities to add to your day that make it more fun and invigorating. Let's face it – in your busy, hectic life, you can all afford a little fun and excitement. The answer to the following questions will propel you forward. They might get you a little uncomfortable, but that is the factor that propels you forward. If the answer to these is yes, it is time to push through and do it. You have the strength with in you to accomplish your dreams. You have the drive to overcome your pain, anxiety, and IBS. You have the desire to propel forward and transform. Just do it. If you say yes to any of these, kick yourself in the butt and push forward. It will be fun and transformational. Are you sick and tired of feeling bloated and crampy? Are you sick and tired of feeling like a whale inside your body? Are you done letting IBS take over your life? Are you done allowing anxiety to stop you? Are you sick of pain controlling your life? Are you ready to have fun and release stress? Are you ready to make yourself the priority? Are you ready to invest in yourself? Alright, awesome. Let's do this.

Let's Get Physical

Let's get physical. "I want to get physical. Let's get into physical. Let me hear your body talk." Lol. I bet you remember that tune from the past. I think it came out in an old movie. Maybe it was *Flash Dance*. I'm not sure lol. My memory wasn't great back then, but the statement definitely stuck. Now, what the heck does that mean? Let's get physical is all about using your body to release stress, emotion, anxiety, and tension. It's about establishing a fun routine that gets your body moving and your voice going.

You spent enough time hiding your feelings, beliefs, and emotions from the world. You were avoiding sharing your opinion, hurt, and pain for far too long. The result of that is our bodies developed these pesky symptoms you desperately want to stop. Our body is expressing anger through pain and symptoms. The secret is to move the energy and emotions within us to allow it to flow. Our bodies are made up of energy, and the energy often gets trapped inside our tissues. That is why you feel tight, tender, and painful spots around your body. There are also tons of toxins and fluids trapped in the fascia of your abdomen that impact your digestive tract. But establishing a routine that gets those muscles moving allows the trapped energy to flow. Establishing a fun vocal routine allows those trapped emotions, worries, and fears to get out too.

I know it sounds strange. I know it seems unrealistic, but it is powerful. Do you remember a time someone told you something that upset you? Did you feel a tightness develop in your body? Maybe your throat got tight. Maybe you took a big gulp and felt a sharp pain in your neck. Maybe your shoulders tensed up. Maybe you got a knot in your back. The location doesn't matter. The fact is you felt your emotion getting trapped inside your body. Your feelings triggered a sensation of pain in your body. Those pesky feelings created a stress response in your body. That pain most likely stuck around for a while. It was there a few hours, days, or weeks.

The more you experience these stressful situations in life and allow them to stay stuck, the worse your pain will become. I'll give you my example, since it is the best way to explain. I spent years of my life keeping my opinions, feelings, and emotions deep inside. Everyone thought I was happy-go-lucky and totally loved going with the flow. But deep inside, I didn't, and I paid for it dearly. As the years passed and I kept keeping every opinion to myself, my throat would tighten, my neck would tense, and my symptoms would accumulate. I was basically strangling my throat every time I kept my opinion to myself. Now, I am not saying to be rude and hurtful towards other people. I am saying to stop being rude and hurtful to yourself. You might not want to stand up for yourself just yet, but you do want to stop feeling crappy and sick all the time.

Here is what I learned. I kept strangling myself and hiding my true feelings, and illness developed. It all started in my neck. The symptoms became overwhelming and worsened more every year. I had chronic neck pain, shoulder pain, thyroid nodules, laryngitis, reflux, and sinusitis. Every single one of those was caused by my inability to express myself. The amount of inflammation that grew in this area was exponential. The symptoms were prevalent. The beautiful thing I learned is that expressing yourself doesn't always have to be vocal. Using the journal activity from Chapter 6 is powerful in releasing those trapped feelings and supporting yourself, too. But your body still needs to use those vocals for self-expression.

Your body still deserves to move, dance, and have fun. That is exactly what this little routine does for you. It is a fun and creative way to release happy hormones throughout your body. It fills you with vibrant energy and empowers your body to heal itself. You can do this anytime. You can do this anywhere. Who cares who is looking? Who cares what they think? The most important person in your life is you. Stop worrying what others think. They are having enough trouble worrying about themselves to really care about you.

Let's get physical with energetic release. You know that exercise and fitness is a great way to reduce stress and enhance physical strength. You know that you should participate in exercise a few times a week, but many of us don't. Most of us tried exercise before and actually felt better while it lasted. Then, something happened that created an obstacle that stopped us. The first thing I will tell you that helps people stick to a routine is to find a partner or support system. If you have a friend that has these same symptoms and deserves to feel better too, then ask them to join you. I guarantee it will make it more fun and create a sense of accountability. Now that you are thinking of a support system, it's time to figure out what do you like to do. Do you like fishing? Hiking? Biking? Dancing? Yoga? Do you like going to a gym? Do you like using workout machines? Do you prefer weight training? Do you like taking classes? Do you like Zumba? Pilates? Tennis?

The activity is irrelevant the fact is, you need to find something that is fun for you. That is the key to keep you motivated, and if you don't have friends to join you, go to a class and make new friends. Create a support system in the environment you choose. Your routine doesn't have to consume your life. But the rule is, you need to get up and get moving. You need to try some activities until you find the ones you enjoy. You need to choose yourself and just do it. Start slow and work up to more activities. Start with thirty minutes to one hour twice a week. Then, work up to at least three days a week. If you work up to five days, then you are a rockstar. It's best if you spread them out a little so your body can recover and rest in between. I prefer Tuesday, Thursday, and Saturday; but maybe for you, it's Monday, Wednesday, and Friday. The schedule doesn't matter but making the commitment does. Schedule your exercise in your calendar. Get ready and prepare for it. If you know you only have time after work on your way to pick up the kids, then be prepared for it. Pack your bag the night before. Take a healthy snack and fluids to drink. Don't allow yourself to make excuses. The more prepared you are, the less likely you are to give up on your dream and achieve your goals. The goal here is to reduce the symptoms of pain, anxiety, and IBS. Get out of your own way and start doing something that releases stress.

Vocalize and Release

Now it's time for the fun stuff. I know it sounds super weird, but vocals are the fun stuff. Do you remember singing, "Whistle While You Work?" As you watched those little dwarfs work hard, helping Snow White clean, do you remember the way you felt? If you don't, then do it now. Stop reading, go find the video on YouTube, and do it. Okay, so, how do you feel now? Was that fun? Did you laugh? Did you smile? Was it silly?

Of course, it was silly. You are a grown up and you just sang a little kids' song. But who the heck cares if it was silly? The fact is, it made you feel good. You want to feel good. The goal now is to sing more and have more fun. My favorite is to do karaoke, record a video, and post it on social. It might be too scary for you to do that. But it's fun. You can record it and then delete it. Just do it. I totally understand the hesitation and fear; the old me was too scared to do it too.

But you can pop in your ear buds and sing while you cook or clean your house. You can turn on the radio and blast your favorite song while you prep your kid's lunches. You can play your favorite music and sing on your way to work. Any of those are super easy. Because you are comfy and safe in your car or home, start there. That is how I started. I am that crazy girl that sings and dances at 7:00 a.m. at a traffic light. I'm that girl that everyone stares at, wondering what she is doing. But I don't care what they think. I am having fun. I am laughing, dancing, and enjoying myself. Those happy, healthy hormones are flowing all over my body. Those happy hormones help your body relax and recover from stress. The question is, are you willing to have fun? Are you willing to sing a little more? Are you willing to be a little silly? One of the things I love to do with my son Lucas is a silly walk. We literally follow each other around the house walking in weird and awkward ways. We have tons of fun and laugh the entire time. We also enjoy dancing and having fun. Have fun with your kids or a girlfriend. Get a little wild and silly. Dancing is easy too. Just turn on the music and go for it. Sing and dance around your house. No one is looking. You can be as silly as you want.

Rest and Recovery

Recovery from exercise is essential. Rest and recovery are important parts of any exercise routine. Your body was designed to move and grove. You need to stay in motion and keep active. You weren't designed to sit at a desk all day. You weren't designed to vegetate on the couch all day. That is why exercise is so important. Exercise and recovery go hand-in-hand to keep your muscles healthy and active. Our muscles need time to stretch and relax. They need a little attention to reduce inflammation, tension, and toxins. You achieve that by establishing a recovery routine.

A recovery routine involves stretching before and after your exercise. That is obvious – you should warm up your muscles before exercise and cool them down after. It is a simple principle that many of us understand but often skip. But don't skip it. Take a few minutes before and after your routine to stretch. Did you know a thorough rest and recovery routine can enhance sleep, relaxation, circulation, and even orgasms? The fact is that as you age, your muscles get tighter; toxins get trapped; and you lose flexibility, range of motion, and actually shrink. Yep, you shrink. Have you ever looked at your grandmother or grandfather? Have you noticed that they are getting shorter? Have you noticed that the less they get around and move, the more trapped they become? Their bodies begin to shrivel and shrink, and immobility is inevitable as these progress.

That is the sad truth of aging. A body in motion is a body in action, but a sedentary body is a body immobile. You don't want to be that forty-year-old that can't walk down the block without getting a cramp in her calf. You don't want to feel trapped inside your body. If you already feel trapped, you want to be free again. But if you sit back and stay stuck, that is exactly what happens. The less you move, the less flexible you become, the more toxins build, and inflammation is stuck. And the more your body shrivels and shrinks as the inflammation gets trapped. I am talking about the muscles, ligaments, and tendons, not the fat.

It's pretty obvious to everyone that weight gain happens with immobility and inactivity but shrinking isn't as obvious. That is a completely different problem, but this exercise and recovery routines will impact weight loss as well. The goal here is not to lose weight, but rather to empower our bodies to become a super stress-fighting machine. A body in motion is capable of achieving anything you dream. The stretching routine I taught myself is not like any other routine I ever saw. It actually promotes circulation and lymphatic drainage. It can be achieved by anyone, but that requires instruction, guidance, and support, which I can offer in a class.

Stretch and Release

Stretching involves using your body or another device to elongate and lengthen your muscles. This simple practice enhances circulation, reduces inflammation, promotes lymphatic drainage and supports your recovery. The best way to understand it is to find a body part that is sore. Yep, a body part that is sore right now. Scan your body and find a place that is tight, sore, or tense. Okay, now is the tricky part, because everyone is different. For me, it is my shoulders and neck. It's time to go on YouTube and find a video to stretch out that sore muscle, or use a stretch you already used before. It might be your shoulders, calf, neck, back, etc.

The location doesn't matter, but you need to find a stretch that feels comfortable for you and try it. My specialty is helping people identify that sore spot, stretch it, and use pressure point massages to relieve it. But I am not there with you. You need to do it alone. Go find that stretch routine and practice it. Once you learn how to stretch that muscle and feel it begin to relieve the tension, I invite you to use the breathing technique you used in Chapter 6. Yep, super weird, but powerful. It's time to combine that stretch with the five-five-five breath. Get in that stretch position and take in a deep breath for a count of five. Now, hold for a count of five and release on an "ahh" for a count of five. Practice a couple of times.

I know it seems silly and weird. But try it. You have nothing to lose but tension and pain. Okay, so now that you tried it, how did that feel compared to just stretching alone? If it didn't feel different, then keep at it. You might need a little more practice. It is perfectly okay, and you need to go at your own pace. The gift of this chapter is that you know you can establish a physical and vocal routine that is fun and invigoration. Now, it's time to keep it in motion. Keep working out two to three times a week. Stretch and recover before and after exercise. Sing and dance to have more fun and release emotions. Add a little stretch and breathing routine to your morning and nighttime schedule. It is best to add this to your bedtime routine, because you will sleep better. I enjoy a little stretch and release before I get up because I am stiff and tight in the morning. Before I get up, I stretch a little in bed. Then, I jump up and head out for the day. Keep moving forward and learning. You are on a path to thrive by releasing your stress regularly. Now, let's learn more about the subconscious mind and pave the way for your unlimited potential to unveil itself.

Energy and Vocals Unleashed

At the beginning of this chapter, I told you about Jenny, who was plagued with fear. She was trapped inside her home almost every day. She desperately wanted to return to work. She worked hard on her transformation and gave herself the attention she deserved. She truly enjoyed the physical release and made new friends at an outdoor Zumba class. She practiced stretching and physical release every day, even when she didn't exercise. But the most fun thing evolved with vocal release. She began to sing all the time. She enjoyed it so much, she started going to karaoke once a week. Her newfound hobby gave her another surprising gift. She met her boyfriend Bob. She was thankful that her new lifestyle empowered her to change. She was grateful to feel vibrant, alive, and free.

CHAPTER 8: AFFIRM YOUR SUCCESS: AFFIRMATIONS, BOUNDARIES, AND PERCEPTION

Affirming the Positive

Milly was a special woman. She loved to help people, but her negative thoughts kept her feeling trapped in her body. Relationships kept leaving her feeling scared, lonely, and unloved. The more her emotions were triggered, the worse she felt. The more trapped she felt, the less she was able to do for herself and others. She became debilitated with pain, fatigue, and bloating. She was so ill that she had to take a leave of absence from her job. Her evolution to success will surprise you, but first, we need to learn about boundaries and perception.

Emotional Rollercoaster

Now, it's time to stop hiding your feelings. It was a struggle for me to develop this skill. I spent forty-one years keeping my opinions, feelings, and beliefs to myself. It was a pattern that took effort and action to unravel and transform. But I realized its significance after challenges and obstacles kept throwing me on my butt. I was sick of the constant rollercoaster of emotions that stopped me dead in my tracks. I was sick of hitting rock bottom over and over again. I was sick of allowing others to make me feel inferior, unlovable, undesirable, unworthy, and invisible. The truth is, it was my perception that was the problem. They were not actually trying to hurt or harm me. They weren't purposefully causing me pain. But my interpretation of the message was skewed. I was getting mixed messages. I was misunderstanding the messages they were sending. It resulted in a multitude of negative emotions inside me. They were all linked to pre-established beliefs from childhood. It took many conversations that triggered an intense response inside me.

This year was truly eye opening as it enlightened me to the importance of perception and boundaries. The powerful thing I learned about relationships is that setting boundaries helps you regain control over the situation. They establish a standard of respect and understanding. It opens a path for you to express your true feelings. But it wasn't easy to achieve. It took time for me to overcome my perception. It took time to see and hear the message with a new filter. This new filter I choose was a filter of love. It took effort on my part to transform those negative feelings and beliefs within me. It was important for me to create a new filter for myself based on love. I began a new practice using affirmations to strengthen this process for myself. I also combined it with hypnosis and meditation, which you already learned about. But using affirmations helped me cement the positive thoughts, new feelings, and beliefs in my mind. You can use affirmations in multitude of ways in your life.

The repetition, reinforcement, and continuity engrain them in your subconscious as you push forward and strive to change.

Affirmations for Success

Affirmations are powerful tools, and you can find them in paintings, plaques, inspirational quotes, podcasts, meditations, and a multitude of other mediums. You can also create unique affirmations for yourself. You can create a powerful mantra for yourself to propel yourself into your transformation and achieve your dreams. It can be as simple as writing it on a Post-It note, buying a magnet, or even creating a word painting. I used every strategy in this book and a multitude of others before I began writing this book. It all began with a little affirmation: "I see, hear, and digest everything with love, joy, and appreciation." A version of this affirmation would pop into my phone as an alarm during my busy day. It all started with the word "love." When it was time for me to write this book and Dr. Angela Lauria. She is the amazing publisher that helped me created this book. In my first lesson, she asked me to pull out a sheet of paper and draw the word that resonated in my body for this book. The word that came to my mind was "love." It was one of my favorite words since childhood. I always use a heart on letters and birthday cards.

I took a few minutes to get creative and colorful with markers. This word art is posted in my kitchen. I see the "love" every day, and it reminds me that this book is a gift of love. It reminds me that I am passing my story on to you with love. Affirmations can come in many shapes and sizes. You can buy them, print them or create them. You might find a cool plaque that says something that brings a smile to your face. If it inspired you in the moment, then buy it. If you can't afford it, then make one. The trick is to find what works for you. One painting I have in my kitchen says, "Love is the greatest gift of all." Another one that is in the entrance of my house says, "Family: Where life begins and love never ends." And if you heard my podcast, "Goddess Unleashed," which launched December 5th, 2019, you know how much the word love means to me. If you ever look at the letters I wrote as a child or the ones I write today, you will see a little heart.

That is simply because love was always so important to me. It was on every letter I wrote. It is on every birthday card I fill out. If I am bored in a class, you will find hearts all over the page. Using love as inspiration, take a moment to write a sentence that expresses your deepest feelings about love. This is what I came up with right now. "Love is nurturing and true and brings more joy and happiness to my life." The affirmation I used for myself today was, "I am free to live the life I dream." You can make your own, find a new one, or use the ones I gave you. Have some fun with it. Go to Google and find some.

There are tons of inspirational quotes, motivational quotes, and affirmations out there. Seek and you shall find – or create your own. Then, put them up everywhere. Set alarms on your phone. Create Post-It notes. Buy a poster for your wall. Whatever it takes to begin to engrain those positive beliefs you desire into your subconscious. Whenever a negative thought comes to mind, use them to transform those thoughts. If your mind says, "I can't do it." Take in a deep breath and think, "I can do it." You are more powerful than you think. Use this simple trick to propel yourself forward. It is important that you see them and read them frequently because the repetition will keep you moving forward. Remember, your inner child wants to stay safe, and your resistance is powerful. Getting out of your comfort zone seems unsafe, which is why the resistance is so formidable and strong.

Don't Let Your Resistance Win

Resistance can stop you in your tracks, but it is a blessing in disguise. It is a curse, because you feel like you can't get past things in the beginning. You feel like you make some progress and fall back down on your butt. But now that you understand perception, boundaries, and affirmations, you are ready to use the resistance to propel you forward. You can take the messages and change things. As you work through each obstacle and challenge, you become stronger and more resilient. You make changes much easier and effectively. You notice the resistance loses its power over you.

September and October were extremely challenging for me, balancing family, nursing, social media, and writing this book. My resistance stopped me from some tasks while I focused on writing this book. It made me feel so overwhelmed with writing on social media or creating videos. It wasn't easy to get out of the creative writing space and enter the live social space. The resistance made me think I could only focus on writing and everything else had to wait. But the truth is, I was ready for more a long time ago. I just needed a nudge in the right direction to get me off my butt. My mentor helped me realize that. Sheena Eizmendiz is the hypnotherapist that trained me. She was watching me evolve and change over the past eight months. She noticed I wasn't on social lately. It took an outsider to make me realize that this part of my journey was also important and valuable to share. Her encouraging words empowered me to shift. That afternoon, I posted a live video after I finished working on a chapter.

Now, I post videos and images every day regardless of the amount of work and writing I am doing. Encouragement came from many coaches and friends along the way. This month in particular, I received so much love to propel me forward. Finally, after almost a year of fighting my resistance, I launched that podcast. Everything in this book is what got me to this point. I wasn't the trapped little girl anymore. I was free to live the life I dreamed. Suddenly, support was coming in all directions. The affirmations, support, and healthy relationships I created helped propel me forward to take action. Everything came together to transform my life. You can transform yours, too. You are more powerful and resilient than you think.

Affirmation Tips:

* Create a colorful mantra image with your personal mantra and save it on the desktop of your phone or computer.   * Write affirmations you like on sticky pads and paste them on your monitor at work.

* Write affirmations on your mirror in the bathroom with a dry erase marker.

* Write affirmations on sticky pads and post them all over your house.

* Set at least three different affirmation alarms into your calendar. Each statement should be different. When the alarm rings, take the time to read it out loud or in your head five times. Your instinct will be to ignore it. Build up to reading it five times. Even it has to wait until you take a break from work. The next time you open your phone, read them before you do anything else.

* Create your personal Mantra on a colorful adult coloring page. Color the page in vibrant colors and stick it somewhere in your house that you will see it every day. When you see it. Read it to yourself five times.

* Use imagery to signal to your brain that it's time for a Mantra. Example: I drink tea every morning at work. Take a moment to think of that cup of tea and tell yourself, "When I see the tea, it is time for my mantra." Your subconscious will begin to identify the tea cup as a signal for you to recite your mantra. Or, even better, buy a mug with an affirmation on it. I have a bunch of inspirational mugs. The one my friends at work got me says,: "Queen of everything."

My Affirmations

Here are some affirmations that transformed my life:
- I am knowledgeable and intelligent.
- I am powerful and true.
- I deserve to be happy.
- I am worthy of more.
- I embrace my unlimited potential to live the life I dream.
- I will accomplish my dreams easily to do, be, and have everything I desire and deserve.
- Love is nurturing and true and brings more joy and happiness to my life.
- Love is the greatest gift of all.
- My family is where life begins and love never ends.
- I thrive under pressure. Everything comes easily and effortless to me.
- My mantra: I help others find their unique happiness and health. This brings me more abundance and prosperity to help more children and families in the community in a meaningful way. I commit to focusing on self-awareness, self-love, and action to care for myself while I help the world around me. I set boundaries to speaking my truth.
- I choose to see everyone and everything with joy and love.
- It's time to fly and be free.
- I see, hear, and digest everything with love, joy, and appreciation.

Boundaries

Boundaries are an important step for you to begin to support your journey and build healthy relationships. Boundaries help other understand your needs and desires. They let others know when enough is enough. They give you the power to control the situation. Trust me, it takes time and practice, but with each boundary you set, the stronger you become. The stronger you become, the more effortless and easier it is to set more boundaries. As the boundaries grow, you become the driver in your relationships. Taking control gives you the power to grow and change. As you grow, you feel safe and supported. The funny thing is that you feel safe and supported in your skin. Your self-esteem and self-love grow because you are finally protecting yourself from those situations, people, and things that used to hurt you. You are finally setting boundaries and making rules for your interactions that keep you safe. Your mind and body are waiting for that feeling of security. Your inner child wants to be protected. You were waiting for your courage to stand up and speak up. Now that you understand perception, affirmations, and boundaries, let me give you an example to help facilitate your journey.

Self-Forgiveness

I had a good friend who appeared to truly care about my feelings. It seemed like he wanted to help. He seemed to be trustworthy and caring. He seemed to want to spend time with me and listen. But after a few months, his true intentions came to light, and the support disappeared. Suddenly, I would text or call, and he was too busy. We would plan coffee or lunch, and he would cancel. Time and time again, a promise was made, and it was never fulfilled. I always gave everything I had. I always promised and delivered, but he never did. Time and time again, I was left frustrated and alone. I felt ashamed and unworthy. I felt unloved and undesirable. I felt so many negative emotions and thoughts that I would fall into a frozen state. Being frozen when you want to take action sucks. You doubt your abilities, you doubt your strength and you lose you drive to push forward.

After months and months of the same scenario, I was sick of being frozen in my tracks. I set a boundary and ended the relationship. I wasn't going to allow another friendship to bleed me dry. There were many relationships over the years that came to an end. This was just another one, but it proved to be trickier than I expected. It wasn't easy to let go. He would pop into my head when a new idea arose in my mind. I desperately wanted to share it. Driving around town would trigger memories too. I would drive by a coffee shop and feel sad. I would see a car that looked like his and get a knot in my stomach. My persistent thoughts and negative beliefs hindered my progress. For months, I pushed through. On the harder days, I worked harder. I wrote letters to him and burned them to say goodbye.

I practiced forgiveness, prayers, and meditations to send him blessings. I prayed and forgave. I was truly forgiving myself for allowing him and others to hurt me. I did this forgiveness practice every day. I had tons of people on my mind during the forgiveness rituals. The days he came into my mind, I prayed again. I blessed him and everyone else in my life. The fact was that the relationship meant more to me than I thought. It took me time to figure out the reason. As I told you before, your subconscious plays tricks on you. It was playing a cruel trick on me.

But in the process, I realized the true pain was in my past. It wasn't from this relationship at all. But without that boundary, I wouldn't figure out the root cause. It was a friendship long lost in my childhood that was causing my heartfelt reaction. I was heartbroken because I lost my best friend, first love, and confidant at age fifteen. He was there for me in my hardest times. He knew everything about me. He supported me through childhood and early teens. We were raised together and grew up together. We were inseparable. But when I met my husband Robert at age fifteen, the friendship became difficult to sustain. I knew that Robert was my true love, and I needed to spend my time with him. That friendship ended a few months after I met my husband, and it was extremely hard to let go. I was sad that this person who shared so much of my past was gone forever. But we were each on a path to new teen love relationships. Little by little, we spoke less. We shared less. It simply ended.

I don't remember any conversation or event that ended things. It just stopped on day. The truth was that when I let him go, I let my memories of my childhood go with him. I lost all the happy and joyful moments we shared because I was so hurt. My stress and emotions caused me to take it out on myself. The emotions that remained left me feeling vulnerable, ashamed, dirty, and broken. That was the little girl inside me that was hurting. My memories disappeared when she closed that door and stayed trapped. But I didn't realize all this pain until I set this new boundary. If I didn't experience the pain again in my current life, I never would connect with it again. Going through this forgiveness process helped me realize those were the feelings that were triggering this reaction.

Those emotions and feeling stayed trapped in my body and my subconscious mind. They continued to hurt me throughout my life. That was truly the friendship I missed, not this one. When I realized that, I added my childhood best friend into my routine. I started to pray for my childhood best friend and let him go, too. Because I realized I never really let go. The little girl inside me was still broken-hearted. She still missed her best friend. She missed having his shoulder to cry on. As the days passed, it got easier. I pushed through; and finally, one day, I forgot that they both existed.

I spent weeks and months without a thought of either of them. I thought I was over the hump. But life is great at sending you a curveball every once in a while. One day, a song played on the radio – "I Forgot That You Existed" by Taylor Swift. At first, I laughed and sang the song. I played it a few days laughing, because it was true. I even told my girlfriend and we both laughed. But playing the song repeatedly, actually brought those painful feelings back. Boom, the thoughts that disappeared from my mind were back. I started the process all over again. I prayed and blessed them both again. I went through all the rituals once more. Poof, they were gone again. Suddenly, things really started to shift. I made big decisions for myself. I began writing again. I began seeing clients and getting unstuck. I began to plan events and follow through, even if no one was there to support me. I began to see the difference in my life. I signed the contract to write this book. I began doing things I never thought were possible. It all started with boundaries and forgiveness. It took me more that twenty-eight years to finally forgive him and myself, because the true pain was in those memories. The true pain was inside my heart. The pain you feel right now is inside your heart. If any emotions or memories came up for you, it's time to embrace the way you feel and let go of the past. That path is set. The secret is at your fingertips now. It's time to forgive yourself. It's time to let go of the past and set yourself free. Are you willing to forgive yourself for the hurt others caused you? Are you willing to practice forgiveness? Are you willing to let go of the past and move forward? Awesome – I am glad you are ready to let go of the past and those pesky symptoms in your body. Let's find out the special blessing I used to forgive myself and let go of the past.

Special Forgiveness Blessing

There was a unique forgiveness process that came to me when I was working on setting that boundary. I was looking for something that really helped me forgive myself for allowing the hurt. I wanted something that blessed them but also supported me. It was time to find something that truly helped me forgive and forget. Well, I never really forgot, because I am writing it here, but I did forgive. It was all thanks to a special forgiveness prayer. It basically landed on my lap when I needed. Because the universe works in mysterious ways. It came to me on my Facebook newsfeed. It came at the perfect time.

I heard about it months before but never tried it. The truth is, you are ready when you are ready. The day I was ready, everything fell into place. I decided to try it. I took a free course and learned about this prayer. I purchased the course that gave me some amazing resources to learn the process. I used meditations, hypnotic intensives, subliminal activations, and everything I learned. *Ho'oponopono*, a Hawaiian prayer, was one of my secret tools. Of course, I added this special gift to everything else I already practiced. I blessed them with the special prayer every day. Each day, the people on the stage changed slightly, but the prayer remained the same. The forgiveness grew stronger within me. This beautiful practice went with me to Hawaii. Every day, when negative emotions began to creep into my mind, I used it. I still use this practice every day. I incorporate it into my routine.

Healthy Relationships

The simple fact is that relationships need to be balanced. There needs to be a give and take from both parties. It isn't healthy for one person to constantly give and the other to only take. If you feel that way, then it's time to take action and protect yourself, because no one can truly protect you from harm. You are your own protector. You need to dig deep and get the courage to express yourself. You need to work to achieve your dreams, passions and desires. You need to feel safe in your skin. That is when you will feel free and powerful. One day, you will finally be free from those relationships that truly hurt you. You can begin to build healthy and strong relationships with those that are truly important to you. You will learn to create boundaries with those that are closest to you.

You will learn to speak your truth and tell them how you feel. You will learn to let go of those emotions that hold you back. The simple truth of the matter is that boundaries help keep you safe. They create a supportive space for you to grow and flourish. It might seem insignificant and unnecessary, but boundaries are the way to emerge from your struggles. Boundaries empower you to propel forward and achieve your dreams. Boundaries allow you to speak your truth. They give you the courage to be heard, loved, and appreciated for everything you are and everything you deserve.

Boundaries are essential if you truly want to tackle your symptoms, IBS, anxiety, and pain, because those pesky symptoms are a sign that you are not happy. They are a sign that you are allowing others to make you feel unsafe, unworthy, unlovable, etc. The more you allow them to impact your inner self, the worse the symptoms become. You know that you don't want those symptoms. You don't want to feel bloated, crampy, and huge. You don't want to feel achy and in pain. You don't want to have a pressure in your chest that makes you panic. You don't want to be stuck in bed when there is a party outside. You don't want to feel trapped inside your body. Get up, dust yourself off, and set those boundaries, because no one will stand up for you unless you stand up for yourself.

Setting Boundaries

There are two types of boundaries: simple and complex. I realized the difference as I worked through creating them in my life. The simple boundaries occur in relationships that aren't so close to your heart, like colleagues, acquaintances, neighbors, or parents at your kid's school. These people are in your life, but they don't play a big role. Your emotions are usually not hurt by them and they don't usually throw you into an emotional rollercoaster. But those are the exact boundaries to set first, because they give you the strength to deal with the truly complex ones.

Then, little by little, you will get the courage to tackle the big ones. You will work up to creating boundaries that are closer to your heart. You will deal with the really complex boundaries. These are necessary because these people are the ones you love. These people were probably in your life an extremely long time. They think they know your feelings, beliefs, and desires, but they really don't. They assume that everything is fine, but it really isn't. These boundaries are the most important because they will impact you every day for the rest of your life. Just keep it simple and start small. Create little boundaries and begin speaking up for yourself. As you begin to feel safer and supported, the courage will grow. You will begin to truly express your feelings, beliefs, and desires. You will be ready to stand up for what you believe all the time, because you will begin to create healthier relationships in your life.

Building Healthy Relationships

Fostering healthy relationships is an important part of evolution and change. You seem to think that your only friends are those you knew forever. Sometimes, those old friends could actually be holding you back. It's important to surround yourself with people that bring you up. People that make you want to strive for more. People that make you want to become a better person. People that truly bring out the best in you. These people motivate you simply with their presence. Going to events or activities with them is easy for you. You feel energized, vibrant, and alive when you are with them. They push you through the hard times and empower you to evolve.

These people are the relationships you need to focus more time on. It doesn't matter if you met them yesterday, last week, or last month. Take time and nurture the relationship if it made a difference in your life. It doesn't matter if you just met them. Plan more time together. If they have a valuable profession that is a great example for you, then join them in a class. Pay for their services and learn from them. Go get coffee, have lunch, or go to a party. There might be a day you have to choose between a family event and time with this person. Choose this person. If they bring value, joy, and fulfillment to your life, they are worth exploring. You are worth it. It's important for you to feel safe and supported. Creating healthy relationships with new people will help you evolve and change. Setting boundaries with old ones keeps you moving forward. The more you change, the more your family and friends will respond. They will become more comfortable with this new version of you.

Accountability Network

Create an accountability network for yourself when you are trying to acquire a new habit. If you want to exercise or meditate, do it with a friend. It is easier to stick to something if you have a friend or mentor by your side. Let them help you accomplish your goals. If you know that you might put your foot down with your family or friends, then call your friend first. Ask them for advice, figure out your plan of action, and let them pump you up before you take action. Then, when you complete that task, they will show you support and praise. They empower you to do the same. Listen and take their advice. Embrace their support and guidance.

My accountability network actually consists of coaches and friends that I met during this journey. They are like minded individuals that experienced similar paths. They understood the struggles I was facing. They supported me through the process. Those are the types of people you want to help keep you on track. Those are the people that will tell you when you are slacking and when you are kicking ass. Those are the people that honestly understand your obstacles because they have overcome many themselves. If you don't have an accountability network, it's time to find one. It's time to find a support system that will keep you accountable in your path to wellness. People that will support you in the good times and the bad. People you can call when you want to cry. People you can call when you want a motivational pep talk. Surround yourself with a multitude, because life keeps everyone busy and it's good to have a few shoulders to lean on.

Relationships Unleashed

At the beginning of this chapter, I presented Milly. She loved everyone so much that she wanted to please them all but forgot to nurture herself. The more she pleased others, the worse she felt. She became plagued with symptoms and discomfort. She created a support system for herself early on in her journey. She focused her transformation on creating boundaries and developing healthy relationships. Her favorite part of the process was her daily forgiveness rituals and affirmations. She had affirmations on her mirror, in her phone, and all over her office. She truly enjoyed the forgiveness ritual. She used the ritual whenever she felt triggered and upset. She forgave everyone and herself. She was grateful that she finally could live her life again without symptoms. She enjoyed volunteering and helping the community. She was grateful for the boundaries she created because they helped her to create meaningful and healthy supportive relationships.

CHAPTER 9: SUCCEED WITH HYPNOSIS – MEDITATION AND SELF-HYPNOSIS

Traumatic Past

My client Betty started with digestive issues as a child. Her constipation was excruciatingly painful. She was sick of all the rectal fissures (tearing of her rectum) from all the straining and hard stool. She hated the hemorrhoids and was sick of the bloating. She was looking to relax more because she had really bad anxiety. Her anxiety usually caused diarrhea during stressful situations. She also had intimacy issues with her partners and felt it was impacting her relationships. She simply wasn't interested in sex. She was in so much pain and discomfort that sex was far from her mind. She had chronic illness and pain in addition to a difficult childhood. She used to enjoy sex but lost that ability long ago. It wasn't only her interest in sex she lost – her body simply didn't respond the same either. She had issues with lubrication and sensations as well. She desperately wanted her libido back.

She recalled events from her childhood that were less than desirable for anyone to experience. But I will explain a little bit just because her secret is always safe with me. The sad truth is that she faced things that no child deserved to endure. Those hurtful things continued to hurt her in her adult life. They impacted her relationships and friendships. She had trouble trusting others and finding a boyfriend. She desperately wanted to marry and have children, but her past made intimacy hard. She met some great partners, but something else always got in the way. After each heartbreak, her physical symptoms got worse and worse.

At that point, her last four breakups took a toll on her body and digestive tract. She was plagued with symptoms that kept her stuck at home. She couldn't go anywhere because her diarrhea was constant. She lost thirty pounds and her doctor told her she needed to decrease stress. She laughed because she had no idea how to do it. But one day, my video popped into her news feed. She said she knew that I could help her. She told me months after that she wasn't sure why she picked up the phone, but she was glad she did. Her symptoms slowly disappeared gradually over the months we worked together. She finally felt some sexual desires returning. She met an amazing man in the process. She was so surprised when her libido popped back into her life. Her body was finally responding how she desired. But her past still got in the way of her intimacy sometimes. I helped her work through her past traumas. It was an essential part of the process to help her feel safe in intimate situations. It also helped create an inner sense of safety for herself.

Betty was abused in her childhood by multiple men in her life. She was physically and sexually abused for years. It is worse than you could possibly imagine. The story brought tears to my eyes when she shared it. She was a strong and powerful woman. She was ready and willing to forgive herself and finally move on. She worked hard to overcome all of that horrific trauma. No child deserves to experience that kind of emotional and physical pain. But she managed to survive it and push through. She worked hard on herself and found her passion for helping others. She began to help victims in the community, and her life began to change. She finally saw the love that was right in front of her. She finally felt better and noticed a friend that was by her side the entire time. He sparked all her desires and interests. She finally found the love she was searching for. She married her best friend. She finally saw the light in her life and felt happy again. Her physical pain improved, and her digestion was amazing. She finally enjoyed food again and didn't feel like symptoms were lurking in the corner. She was free to go to parties and events again. She was free to have fun again. She thanks me to this day. She was most grateful for her new life because she found love. They created a beautiful family and she finally had everything she wanted and deserved. She pops in for sessions in her fun-filled life just to stay on track. She was amazed that in search of a solution for her symptoms, she found so much more than she expected.

Emotional Turmoil

Lilly had a traumatic past. She experienced things in her childhood that no one should endure. She was suffering from chronic pain, fatigue, and frequent vaginal infections. She knew her pain was related to her past. She had some vague recollection of abuse but really wanted to understand it better. She wanted to enjoy sex and intimacy more with her husband. But her traumatic past was keeping her feeling stuck. She wanted to uncover the secrets from her past and finally overcome them. She transformed her life in a multitude of ways. But before we can talk about her evolutions, it's time to understand the emotional root.

The Emotional Root

Now that you understand the physical root cause of IBS and the herbs that can reduce inflammation and cell damage, it's time to talk about your emotions. The emotional root cause of our symptoms goes deep into our past. Our beliefs, feelings, and emotional responses were established well before you could even understand them. This emotional foundation takes us to our childhood. All of this emotional programming occurred before the age of eight. It involves all your pre-established feelings, thoughts, and beliefs that impact your current day life. It includes but is not limited to any unresolved traumas, worries, and fears that were engrained in your subconscious during those early years. These tricky worries, fears, and traumas trigger our emotional reactions and behaviors throughout our lives.

These feelings and beliefs were created at a time in our lives when you were learning to cope with the environment, people, and world around you. Many of these reactions were established and engrained in our subconscious without a conscious understanding. Most of them are feelings, beliefs, and emotions you truly don't believe, accept, or agree with. Those beliefs, thoughts, emotions, and feelings impact our daily lives hiding in our subconscious every second. They impact every decision you make whether you are aware of it or not. When you make a decision that goes against your true desires and beliefs, your body responds. This emotional reaction erupts in your body with or without your awareness. They are evident in your body through symptoms, pain, illness, and disease.

I know it sounds crazy. This seems weird and impossible. I thought so, too, until I started digging deep into my emotional past using hypnosis. I knew that my anxiety began early in my childhood and progressively worsened over my life span. At this point, I was in my forties and emotional stress was still getting the better of me. Even though I incorporated nutrition, fitness, and alternative treatments into my life, stress was still triggering anxiety and IBS. It was also impacting my life and experiences. I desperately wanted to help people heal their physical and emotional pain, but fear kept stopping me in my tracks. It was a constant rollercoaster trying to get my business off the ground. I would take a few steps forward and then revert right back to my old ways. I would begin to write and share my thoughts on my blog, but confrontations or conversations would set me on an emotional rollercoaster.

This constant emotional rollercoaster happened in my life and the lives of my patients. I could clearly see that there was an underlying issue that addressing the physical root was not resolving. My emotions brought on IBS, migraines, illness, disease, and extreme physical pain. I was desperate to learn exactly why I had so much trouble expressing my feelings. Why was it so hard for me to tell people I disagreed with something? Why did everyone think I was happy-go-lucky? Why did everyone expect me to go with the flow no matter what? Why was I okay living like this all my life? Why was a sitting back and letting people take advantage of me? Why did loud, emotional confrontations make me want to hide? Why did I continuously get flare ups of my symptoms after these highly emotional moments? Why? Why? Why?

This sets the foundation for my understanding of the importance of addressing the emotional root. I decided to undergo hypnosis to find the answers. There were some pretty surprising things I unveiled. I finally realized why my memory was so bad and I couldn't recall much of my past. I understood that I developed this protective coping mechanism in my childhood that actually went against my personal desires. I learned at a young age to hide and stay quiet. I learned that it was safer if I kept my feelings to myself. I chose to live this way since a young age. My body didn't like it one little bit.

My body was so against this hiding that I developed digestive issues, constipation, and body pains in childhood. Guess what? It created inflammation and stress inside my body, which was the physical root of the problem. But the emotional component added extra stress on my mind and memory. A body and mind that is under stress has trouble retaining information because of the constant assault stress had on them. Thus, my memory sucked. I chose to sit back and let people walk all over me. I allowed every decision to be made for me. I lived this way my entire life and my body was not happy with it. The simple fact is that hypnosis helped me uncover the beliefs from the past that I was ready to rewrite. It unlocked the secrets of my mind to give me the strength to move forward and leave the past behind.

Hypnosis empowered me to work on each pesky belief I didn't agree with until I saw shifts in my life. The details of the sessions aren't as important as the end result. The past is in the past, and it unveiled an opportunity to change, grow, and evolve. I was ready to truly change my life and help people, but until hypnosis, I couldn't get those pre-established beliefs out of my way. Those engrained negative beliefs and emotions wouldn't let me live the life I wanted. I couldn't stop those negative feelings, beliefs, and emotions from impacting my life no matter how much I tried. It impacted me in my personal life, social life, and career every day. Without digging into my past to find the emotional root cause, I never truly impacted the physical reaction.

Hypnosis helped me access those negative beliefs and reframe them in my subconscious. After that eye opening experience, the final steps in my process finally began to evolve. Overcoming the issues from my past unveiled the opportunities the future had in store. The deep understanding of my actual beliefs helped me create a routine to transform those negative thoughts into action.

You already understand physical and emotional stressors caused symptoms in the body. To impact these physical and emotional stressors, you need to go to the root of both of them simultaneously. That is the fastest way to truly reduce your symptoms, illness, and disease. Tackle the stress at the emotional and physical root to thrive in your life and achieve your unique wellness. Now that you truly understand to physical and emotional root, take in several deep breaths and think about it all for yourself. What is your medical history? What are your current symptoms? How does thinking about these symptoms make you feel? Do any emotions come up? Do any conversations make your symptoms worse? Do certain relationships trigger your symptoms? Just close your eyes and breath. Think about it. Something will come up in your mind. Now, it's time to learn a little more about building a nutritious foundation for healing.

The Goal Is in Sight

Let's face it, you are all familiar with pain. You experienced pain in your life. Some people experience much more pain than others, but the fact is, you want it to stop. You suffer from emotional and physical pain on a regular basis. You want to leave the pain behind and live the life of your dreams. You want to feel fulfilled, happy, and alive. You want to feel wanted, needed, and loved. You want to feel supported, safe, and nurtured. But there is one critical part of you that controls every aspect of your life, whether you like it or not. It is the part of you that stops you from speaking up for yourself. It stops you from going after that amazing job. It stops you from going up to that attractive person and starting a conversation. It happens to everyone at one moment or another.

Some people experience it more prevalently. I've said it before, and I will say it again. Our pesky subconscious mind controls the path to our future. It is the part of our bodies that is destined to hold us back because it fears change. It desperately wants to stay safe. Being safe usually means staying stuck. Unless you actively transform those negative feelings and beliefs that hold you back, you will never truly accomplish your dreams. If you allow your mind to keep you safe, you will never achieve your ultimate hopes and desires. This chapter is going to be different from the rest. It will give you meditation and hypnosis scripts. These scripts will begin to change those engrained negative beliefs about yourself in a unique way. This will propel you forward to accomplish your dream and overcome your IBS. The thing I noticed in this last year of transformation was that my fears created my resistance to change. The resistance can stop you dead in your tracks. It can stop your progress completely. The fear can make you feel like you are on a constant rollercoaster. It feels like life is sending you an overwhelming number of obstacles and challenges.

The fact is, our lives will continue to send obstacles and

challenges our way. It wouldn't be fun if life was easy. If you had everything you dreamed of every moment of every day, it would be boring and uneventful. Eventually, it would feel dull and monotonous. The obstacles and challenges actually empower us to keep changing and shifting. They push us to become better versions of ourselves. Tackling those fears and worries that hold us back is essential for that evolution. That is exactly why you need to tackle that subconscious if you want to stay in motion. Trust me, I tried to avoid this for years. That is why it took me seven years to get to where I am today. No one deserves to suffer for seven or ten or twenty years with pain, symptoms, illness and disease. No one deserves to feel trapped inside their bodies. That is where I was most of my life trapped inside a body filled with emotions and pain. I can tell you no one deserves to live that way. No one should have to feel scared, ashamed, and doubtful of their potential. No one should feel trapped, unworthy, undesirable, and ashamed. Yet, I felt it every day of my life. But it all unraveled as I transformed my subconscious mind to unveiled my ultimate potential through hypnosis.

Transform the Subconscious

The goal here is to create a routine that stops your mind from throwing you off course. There are two different strategies that I use every day to work on my subconscious blocks, emotions, and feelings. These strategies are meditation and hypnosis. Affirmations are also an important part, which I discussed earlier. There are different types of meditations, but the principle is simple. Meditation is a time to quiet your mind, calm your thoughts, and refocus your attention on your inner self. It is a peaceful time to relax and re-center your thoughts. Meditation is an amazing gift to start off your day feeling motivated, energized, and alive. It is an awesome tool to use when you feel stressed, anxious, overwhelmed, or worried. If your body is giving you signs that you are feeling stressed during the day, take a few minutes to quiet your thoughts through meditation.

I understand the hesitation and fear. I didn't think I could sit quietly with my thoughts either. After all, my mind just kept going constantly. From the moment my eyes opened until I drifted off to sleep, my mind was always racing. Worrying about the kids: What I need to do next? What bills I do I need to pay? What should I do about my chronic pain? And I also spent hours worrying about "what if:" What if I answered that question wrong? What if Betty was mad at me because I just said no? What if I failed that test? What if I fell off the bicycle? It was impossible to stop the constant negative banter in my head without hypnosis and meditation. Now, I ask you this. What if you don't do anything about your IBS right now? What happens if you continue to allow people to step all over you? What if you don't go after that man you like? What if you don't get out of your own way and move forward? What if your anxiety and stress continue to grow?

The answer is, you stay stuck in the exact situation you are trying to avoid. You will stay hiding inside your house because your stomach is bloated and crampy. You will spend hours at the doctor because your pain, diarrhea, and cramps are overwhelming. You will feel overwhelmed and anxious over and over again. Confrontations will continue to trigger your symptoms. Relationships will continue to make you feel unsafe, and symptoms will emerge. The pattern won't stop just because you want it to. You need to take *action* and move forward. You need to transform the *subconscious* thoughts that hold you back. You need to stop that *negative Nancy* in your head. You need to change your thoughts to change your future. That is exactly what hypnosis did for me.

Hypnosis unlocked the little lies that my *negative Nancy* kept reciting in my head: "You aren't good enough," "You aren't smart enough," "You aren't knowledgeable enough," "You should be ashamed of yourself," "You should be guilty you did that." "You are undesirable." "You are not beautiful." Trust me I understand negative thoughts deeply. N*egative Nancy* also filled me with fear, self-doubt, shame, guilt, and worry. It wasn't easy to push myself to see a therapist. It wasn't easy to work on those emotions and feelings, but it was worth it. Because if I didn't do the work, I wouldn't be writing this book. I was too scared to speak my truth. I was too scared to tell my story. I was too fearful of being judged. I realized that transforming those pesky negative thoughts was going to take action, practice, and persistence.

The most effective way to transform things is to get a hypnotist or hypnotherapist like me to develop a personalized hypnosis program for you. This will cultivate a unique hypnosis to tackle your unique fears, obstacle, or challenge. This is the secret to truly unveiling your ultimate potential and impacting your health and your life. These challenges, obstacles, and fears will change over time. It is possible to download and listen to things on the internet. I did face-to-face hypnosis. I took multiple courses that offered hypnosis audios. I did them all, and the ones that are most effective and efficient are the individualized sessions created for you. But truly, the most important factor is your investment in your personal development. When you choose to make an investment in yourself, it impacts your subconscious. This monetary contribution empowers your pesky subconscious to actually put more effort into the process. If you spend $5,000 on a course, you will work much harder at accomplishing it and completing it than if it was free. One of the most impactful hypnosis courses was by Dr. Joe Vitaly. It is an amazing course about hypnosis that using the principles of love and forgiveness. This little prayer helped me develop my strategies of forgiveness.

Let's face it: it isn't easy for us to forgive others. You let those negative feelings and emotions fester with in you. You dwell on the past, and it stops you from moving forward. The sad truth is that if you don't forgive, you are actually hurting yourself. The other person isn't feeling the pain and symptoms. They aren't experiencing the cramping, stomach pain, and bloat. They aren't suffering for days and weeks, trapped inside their bodies. But you are, and that is the problem. The reason forgiveness is an essential part of my program is because it is the last phase I needed to propel forward. I needed to stop blaming myself for the hurt others caused in my life. I needed to stop using those negative emotions and thoughts on myself. This special prayer gave me that. I am not saying you need to be religious or go to church. I am not saying anything of the sort, actually. I am just saying that these powerful words and this powerful ritual actually help you cut the cords of pain that are holding you back.

It helps you forgive others, but it's true power means you forgive yourself. The words are so simple that it inconspicuously has this huge effect on your life. It reinforces self-love in your subconscious mind. You will see that I use these words in meditations, hypnosis, and other self-loving practices. The words are so simple, it will appear like they are too simple to be effective. But the opposite is true. The words are: "I am sorry. Please forgive me. Thank you, and I love you." These little words helped me forgive myself for allowing others to hurt me. It allowed me to forgive myself for keeping all those negative feelings trapped inside me all my life. It gave me freedom from my past by letting go of the relationship and moving on. I used it to enhance my healing and build stronger relationships. It empowered me to set more boundaries. Then, you finally achieve your dreams and desires because you are truly safe and supported in your skin.

Hypnosis Unveiled

Lilly was plagued by her traumatic past. She wanted to uncover the secrets from her past to transform her future. She was sick of her pain and symptoms. She also wanted to connect deeper with her husband but knew her trauma was holding her back. She worked on her transformation daily. She was so dedicated that she went above and beyond. She listened to her personalized hypnosis sessions every day. She loved her morning and evening meditations. She was pleasantly surprised when her libido re-emerged. She was most thankful that she finally didn't feel trapped inside her body anymore. She finally understood her abuse was not her fault. She was able to move and live the life she deserved. She was most grateful for her spectacular orgasms. She couldn't believe that transforming her mind through hypnosis and lifestyle adjustments made such drastic changes in her life.

Your Meditations and Self-Hypnosis

But the free stuff can help you begin the transition, so here are some meditation and hypnosis scripts that you can read to yourself to work on that subconscious mind. It is even better if you record yourself reading these scripts slowly and play them over and over again. Yep, super weird, I know. But super powerful to hear yourself speaking positive, uplifting thoughts and visions in your ear. Get on the highway to your future. Get on the bandwagon to change your life. Take out your voice recorder and read these scripts for yourself. Trust me, I am here if you are ready to *invest* in your transformation and want additional support. I enjoy using background noise in the recordings for added calming effect.

It will be amazing if you do that for the meditation. Continue to use the background noise during the affirmation portion of the meditation. Hypnosis scripts can be fun to record and replay. You can go to my website and make your own recordings using the hypnosis scripts. The easiest option is to download my recordings, which were created as a resource for this book. Just take some time now to read these scripts and record them. When you see, this is an anchor. It is used to anchor the positive emotions and feelings with your new self. Use the cues to use a noise in the recording to reinforce the anchor in your subconscious. It can be a bell, sound bowl, or chime. It doesn't matter what you choose – just use something. Choose one meditation a week and listen to it morning and night or find another meditation you enjoy and listen to it. Choose one hypnosis a week and listen to it at least once a day. If you want to access these unique recordings and make it easier on yourself, just go to my website and download them (dianevich.com/resources). I will see you in the next chapter.

Hypnosis and Meditations Scripts

Morning Meditation

I Invite you to close your eyes and relax. There is nothing to do. Nothing to think about. That's right. You are completely relaxed and calm. I invite you to imagine you are standing on a beach with the warm, soothing sand on your feet. As you glance into the horizon, you see the sun is slowly rising. The warm orange glow is soothing and relaxing. As the sun rises, you feel more energized and vibrant. That's right – with each second that passes, you feel more alive.

The warmth of the sun begins to tickle your skin. The warmth against your skin is soothing and comforting. The orange glow is growing more vibrant in the sky. As the sun fully emerges, you feel a sense of resilience throughout your body. You feel strong, powerful, and energized. That's right. As you peacefully imagine yourself looking at the horizon in the distance, the resilience grows stronger within you. Now as you settle your thoughts and calm your mind, continue to repeat this centering thought. "I am resilient and vibrant. I am resilient and vibrant. I am resilient and vibrant. I am resilient and vibrant. I am resilient and vibrant. I am resilient and vibrant. I am resilient and vibrant. I am resilient and vibrant. I am resilient and vibrant. I am resilient and vibrant." Amazing – all those centering thoughts are serving you now in your subconscious.

You feel vibrant energized and alive. You are ready to forgive and let go of the past. I invite you now to create a stage on the beach. This stage is beautifully decorated with beautiful flowers and vines. The sun is shining brightly on the stage. It is warm peaceful and inviting. As you take in a deep breath and exhale, I invite you fill the stage with anyone that came to your mind today. Invite everyone to that stage. Anyone that is with you mentally, physically, or spiritually. That's right – watch them all walk upon the stage and face you. I invite you now to take in a deep, long breath and hold briefly. Perfect. That's right.

Now, slowly release your breath. As you release, notice the sunlight is beaming its warm, loving glow on you. It is shining its loving light upon you and everyone on the stage. You feel this warmth comforting you from head to toe. You feel the warmth traveling down your body, from your head to your toes. That's right – you are completely relaxed and comfortable. The warmth is giving you more strength and resilience.

You feel joy filling up your heart as the warmth penetrates your body. You are completely filled with pure loving light from your toes to your head. That's right. It is warm, soothing, and comforting. I invite you now to begin to send love and forgiveness to everyone on the stage. As you look at everyone on the stage, repeat these words in your head or say them. It's completely perfect however you choose. "I'm sorry, please forgive me, thank you, I love you. I'm sorry, please forgive me, thank you, I love you. I'm sorry, please forgive me, thank you, I love you. I'm sorry, please forgive me, thank you, I love you. I'm sorry, please forgive me, thank you, I love you. I'm sorry, please forgive me, thank you, I love you. I'm sorry, please forgive me, thank you, I love you. I'm sorry, please forgive me, thank you, I love you." That's right. Just like that.

As you repeat those words one last time, you see a glowing light from the sun shining down upon everyone on the stage. It is glowing and healing them completely, from head to toe. That's right. With all the love inside your heart, I invite you to say those words one last time. "I'm sorry, please forgive me, thank you, I love you." Now, the loving light leaves them all glowing brightly. They are safe, peaceful, and serene. Your blessings and forgiveness left them completely healed. It's time to pick up the cords that connect you to everyone on this stage. Pick them all up. That's right. Just like that. Use a beam of pure, loving light to cut the cord. As you cut the cord, you send one last loving blessing to everyone on that stage.

As the cord is cut, everyone begins to disappear from the stage. That's right. Just like that. You watch them disappear with a deep, loving glow. All these beautiful blessings supported you and everyone on the stage. This process forgave you and everyone on that stage. You are completely relaxed, peaceful, and serene. You feel invigorated with a joyful and happy energy flowing throughout your body. That's right. In a moment, you will awaken with all those happy emotions flowing freely within you.

Now, I invite you to take in five deep, long breathes to finish the process. That's right. Breathe deeply. Hold for a moment. That's right. Breath in deeply for a count of five and hold briefly before you release. As you finish the last breath, you open your eyes. You are completely relaxed, peaceful, and serene That's right. As you exhale that last long breath you feel vibrant, loved, and alive. You open your eyes to live a blessed and happy day.

Evening Meditation

I invite you to close your eyes and relax. That's right. There is nothing to do. Nothing to think about. You simply breath, relax, and let go. That's right. Just like that. You are completely relaxed and calm. With each breath, your body is sinking deeper and deeper into the bed. Each breath you take relaxes you deeper and deeper. I invite you to imagine yourself hanging in a hammock on the beach. The cool summer night's breeze is tickling your skin. As the sensation travels throughout your body, you become more relaxed and settled. That's right, just like that. You are floating in that hammock and gently swing in the wind. The breeze is relaxing you deeper and deeper. As you glace towards the ocean, you notice a bright, glowing moon in the purple sky. The sight of the moon is calm and inviting. The simple sight of the moon makes you sink deeper and deeper into the bed.

The gentle breeze is relaxing and soothing. The orange glow is growing more vibrant and brilliant in the sky. Now, as you settle your thoughts and calm your mind, continue to repeat this centering thought. "I am peaceful and calm. I am peaceful and calm. I am peaceful and calm. I peaceful and calm.

I am peaceful and calm. I am peaceful and calm. I am peaceful and calm. I am peaceful and calm. I am peaceful and calm. I am peaceful and calm. I am peaceful and calm." Amazing – all those centering thoughts are serving you now in your subconscious for deeper peaceful sleep.

You are ready to drift off to sleep soon. That's right. You are so peacefully relaxed that you will drift off easily to sleep. You will have a restful night's sleep. That's right. Before you drift off, it's time to let go of anything that bothered you today. Anything that made you upset or worried. You are ready to forgive and let go. That's right, just like that. You release and let go of anything that bothered you. That's right.

I invite you now to create a stage on the moon lite beach. This stage is beautifully decorated with intricate delicate flowers. The warm glow of the moonlight is gently lighting up the stage. As you take in a deep breath and exhale all those things you want to let go from today come instantly to your mind. That's right. All those feelings, emotions and thought pour onto the stage leaving you peaceful, calm and relaxed. That's right. Now, you invite anyone to the stage that came to your mind today. Anyone that is with you mentally, physically, or spiritually. The stage is glowing in the moonlight. The warm, purple sky is peaceful and serene. That's right. Watch them all walk upon the stage and face you.

I invite you now to take in a deep, long breath and hold briefly. That's right. As you slowly exhale, release any negative feelings, thoughts, or beliefs that stayed behind. That's right. You are ready to let it go. Letting go of everything that no longer serves you. Just like that. As you release, you notice the moonlight and stars are beaming on you. The moon is shining its loving light upon you and everyone on the stage. You feel its warmth comforting you from head to toe. You feel the warmth traveling down your body, from your head to your toes. That's right.

You are completely relaxed and comfortable. The warmth is filling you with a sense of peace, calm, and serenity.

You feel resilient and strong. You feel joy filling up your heart as the warmth penetrates your body. You are ready to begin your evening with love and forgiveness. As you look at everyone on the stage, repeat these words. Say them in your head or verbalize them. It's completely perfect however you choose. That's right. "I'm sorry, please forgive me, thank you, I love you. I'm sorry, please forgive me, thank you, I love you. I'm sorry, please forgive me, thank you, I love you. I'm sorry, please forgive me, thank you, I love you. I'm sorry, please forgive me, thank you, I love you. I'm sorry, please forgive me, thank you, I love you. I'm sorry, please forgive me, thank you, I love you. I'm sorry, please forgive me, thank you, I love you." That's right. Just like that.

As you repeat those words one last time, you see a glowing moonlight is shining down upon everyone on the stage. It is glowing and healing them completely, from head to toe. That's right. With all the love inside your heart, I invite you to say those words one last time. Let go of everything from today, leaving you peaceful, calm, and serene. That's right. Now, I invite you to take in a deep long breath. That's right. Hold it briefly before you release it slowly. Now repeat the phrase one last time. "I'm sorry, please forgive me, thank you, I love you." Now, you see the loving light is glowing gently upon everyone. It's time to pick up the cords that connect you to everyone on this stage. Pick them all up and use a beam of pure, loving light to cut the cord. As you cut the cord, you send one last loving blessing to everyone on that stage. That's right. You watch them disappear into the deep, loving glow. A sense of peace and calm fills your body.

Now, I invite you to take in five deep, long breathes to finish the process. That's right. Breath in and hold briefly five more times. Just like that. As you exhale that last long breath, you feel completely relaxed and calm. Focus on your breathing now. You are slowly breathing in and out. That's right. You are peaceful, calm, and relaxed, and ready for a long night's sleep. You are simply relaxing deeper and deeper into your bed. As the words slowly disappear, you will drift off easily and effortlessly. That's right. You are ready to drift off into a deep and restful night's sleep.

Releasing Self-Doubt from Your Gut

I invite you to close your eyes and settle into your chair. That's right, just relax and let go. Every noise you hear, including the sound of my voice, will allow you to relax deeper and deeper. That's right. You are completely calm and relax.

You are so relaxed, you are sinking ten times deeper into a state of peace, calm, and serenity. Each slow breath relaxes you deeper and deeper into your chair. That's right. With each breath, you sink deeper and deeper into a state of complete relaxation. Now, I invite you to breath and hold briefly. That's right. As you exhale slowly, you feel your body relax deeper and deeper. I invite you to take a deep breath. Perfect, just like that. Breath in, filling up your lungs with air. That's right. Now, hold it a few seconds. Amazing. Feel your exhale as you release it slowly out of your mouth. Notice how your body relaxes more and more with each breath.

As you breathe, your mind becomes calm and quiet. There is nothing to do, nothing to think about. You are simply breathing relaxing and letting go. Your muscles are loosening and relaxing more and more as you breathe. That's right. Now, I invite you to scan your body and notice any tension that remains. Allow your body to let it go with your breath. That's right. You release and relax and let it all go. The more you breath slowly, the more your body relaxes. That's right. The relaxation is flowing freely everywhere throughout your body. That's right. I invite you to take another deep breath. As you exhale, imagine every last bit of tension is melting away from your body. You are fully relaxed, calm, and serene. That's right, just like that.

Now, I invite you to imagine a shower in front of you. It is a huge, white shower with beautiful, intricate tiles on the walls. The designs have butterflies and flowers in delicate colors accentuating the walls. The walls are glistening with moisture. It looks so peaceful and inviting to you. It has a large shower head on the roof. The water flows gently and reminds you of a waterfall. That's right. It looks so relaxing and inviting that you step a little closer. As you walk inside and feel the flow of water trickling down your body, you notice more water is flowing from all directions. That's right. Water is flowing from the walls with a pink glow. The water begins to flow all over your skin. It is gentle and soothing. That's right.

The water is warm and soothing all over your skin. The flow of the water is calming and relaxing. Slowly, the pressure of the water is increasing around you. The water is starting to gently apply a slight pressure on your skin. It is focusing its intense pressure on those areas of your body that you are self-conscious about. All those areas where you feel you are too big, undesirable, unwanted, or unlovable. There is a spout right in front of your belly gently but firmly massaging your stomach. That's right. Its gentle massage is releasing any negative thought, feelings, and emotions. The gentle massage is soothing and warm. That's right. It is massaging that tender and sore spot in your tummy. It is soothing all the discomfort you were feeling. That's right. Your tummy is calm, peaceful, and relaxed. As the water continues to massage you, you notice you're feeling more relaxed and calmer. All those negative feelings, thoughts, and emotions are flowing freely from your body.

You are more peaceful, calm, and relaxed. As you look down at your belly, you notice that your boated belly is shrinking. Those fears and worries that were bothering you are washing away down the drain. That's right. It is soothing, yet forceful. The warm, soothing water is leaving your stomach peaceful, calm, and serene. You notice the water is allowing those fears and stressors to melt away from your body. That's right. You feel those areas are slowly diminishing. That's right. That pesky bloating that no longer serves you is disappearing before your eyes. With each slow breath, you feel more peaceful and calmer.

Your mind is realizing those old stressors don't serve you anymore. You smile as you watch them drain out of your body.

Those stressors are leaving your mind and your body. That's right. There is nothing to worry about or fear now. The soothing water relaxes you deeper and deeper. Those stressors are all circling down the drain and disappearing. That's right, just like that. Let them go. Those stressors don't define you. They are the old you. Now that all those stressors left your body, that emotional and physical pain in your tummy is disappearing as the water flows. Those negative feelings don't serve you anymore. They are the old you. All those negative emotions were part of the old you. You see them circle the drain and disappear. All those stressors disappear. That's right, just like that.

They don't serve your body anymore because you are safe and protected here. Those stressors were part of the old you. You are safe and supported in your own skin. You feel completely calm, peaceful, and serene. That's right. The water is slowing down. That's right. The flow is slowly stopping. The gentle flow of water slowly begins to stop. The water trickles its last few drops of warm liquid on your body. You feel a sense of joy and happiness emerging throughout your body. It is rising from your feet up to your head. You watch the last drops of water circle down the drain. As you slowly step out of the shower, you see yourself in the mirror. You are beautiful, vibrant and alive. That's right. I invite you to see the New You in the mirror as you step towards it – this New You.

You feel beautiful, calm, peaceful and relaxed. You feel safe and supported in your own skin. You slowly walk out of the shower and watch the water evaporate off your skin. You look at yourself in the mirror and you look amazing. This is the New You. This is the powerful version of yourself that you desired. It is the new you. It is the strong, confident, and resilient you. Your skin is glowing, and the beauty is radiating off your body. You love yourself deeply. That's right. You love this New You. You are going to do everything in your power to support this fabulous New You. You love this New You so much that this self-love routine becomes easy and effortless. That's right. You do everything to support your body easily and effortlessly. You eat the

CHAPTER 10: HOLISTIC HEALTH – ENERGY MEDICINE AND YONI HEALTH

Yoni Pain Revealed

Missy experienced a traumatic sexual experience in her teens. It left her terrified of intimate situations and plagued by pain. She suffered from pain, IBS, and fatigue. She desperately wanted to improve her sexual experiences with her new boyfriend. Her transformation will surprise you, but first, it's important to understand the truth about pain.

Understanding a Deeper Truth About Our Pain

It's not always easy for people to let go of the stress and challenges life brings. It can sometimes be a complex process to overcome your obstacles on a daily basis. But for women, the truth is that it's even harder. It is ten times harder because women are highly emotional beings. You take your emotions and feelings to a level that men just can't comprehend. They simply don't understand the way we think or feel. People don't understand the way your body works in response to stressful situations. They have trouble connecting with your deepest, darkest dreams and desires because you tend to hide them from view.

You obscure your reality in such a way that it makes it almost impossible for a man to understand and connect with you. All this happens because you were born with an emotional higher power. I'm not saying you are better than men in any way; just that you have some unique attributes that can either hinder you or propel you forward. You were born with a unique gift inside your body. You were given the blessing and power to carry another human within you. You may not all choose to live the life of motherhood, but your body was designed for it. But with this beautiful gift comes additional challenges and obstacles that men will never truly understand, because they can't live in your body and walk in your shoes.

You face hormonal imbalances that make your emotions go haywire. These emotions can be so intense sometimes that you might pick a fight with a complete stranger for no apparent reason. They can also impact you in daily interactions and impact your relationships. You became accustomed to those hormonal fluctuations as a normal part of life. After all, it began with the gift of menstruation. You also get physical symptoms every month that can be debilitating and excruciating. Not everyone gets this regularly, but those that do experience menstrual or hormonal issues understand the pain. It can literally stop you in your tracks and keep you in bed for days. I was one of those teens that couldn't move from the intense menstrual cramps and bleeding.

Oh, such a blessing, right? When you experience all these symptoms, it makes you wish you could make it disappear. But really, your gift is a blessing once you unleash your feminine energy and inner strength. You just haven't figured out why or how yet. But in my journey through healing, I learned that our emotional and physical pain doesn't have to be so severe and debilitating. It doesn't have to stop you from pleasure, and it sure as heck isn't there to create havoc in your life. But there are ways to tap into your natural feminine gifts to create a flow that frees you from the hormonal rollercoaster, pain, and symptoms. Yes, you have hormones. Yes, sometimes they might be imbalanced.

You should always go to the doctor and make sure there are no serious health concerns. But you don't need to spend countless hours at specialists looking for answers without taking action for yourself. I believe it's essential for women to go to their annual gynecologic exams. Also, get your mammogram every year when it's due. However, I am saying that you can get your feminine energy to flow in a way that supports your emotional and physical health. Trust me, it took me years to find it. After all, I was chronically inflamed and had no libido since my mid-thirties. Sex was a chore, and I was too exhausted and in pain to initiate it. But once my body began to heal, this little spark happened that surprised me. The first time it happened was on a vacation with my husband. I spent years with no real interest in sex, but on vacation, I was so relaxed and well-rested that orgasms came easily. This particular orgasm scared me, even though it was amazing.

I was already changing my lifestyle to reduce inflammation, and things were beginning to awaken my libido. This particular night, after a glass of wine and a delicious vegan chocolate cake, that libido got superpowers. My orgasm went on for hours. Simply the breeze from the fan would trigger me deeper into an orgasm. It was amazing and excruciating at the same time. But after that day, the libido I was lacking was more prevalent, and I felt calmer throughout the month. I noticed the more sex I had. the less bloating, cramping, and hormonal shifts I felt. Progressively, this continued to increase over the years. This little, unique gift slowly began to enhance my life in other ways. It enhances your sacred sexual energy and pleasure centers. This unique gift is yours and yours alone. Men also hold stress in their genitals and rectum. They also hold trauma and hardships there too. This routine is beneficial for them as well, even though they don't have a Yoni. Kegels are universal and will benefit both parties. But this book focuses on women, because I truly deeply understand their healing process because I experienced.

Your Yoni

This powerful energy-flowing machine allows your body to relax, unwind, and disconnect in a special way. It all starts with a little secret you didn't know about your vagina. Let's call it by its sacred sexual name instead of the medical term: your Yoni. Yep, that's right, your Yoni makes you special and unique. Here is the little-known secret that stops us in our tracks and causes the emotional and physical rollercoaster. That rollercoaster sends us on a tangent towards symptoms. Our yoni, which was created to birth a child, was made with a slight flaw. Overcoming this little flaw is possible even in women with a traumatic past. I say that because I saw it time and time again.

Women who were abused, raped, or emotionally abused emerged from their trauma with a unique feminine energy and orgasmic power that others simply can't understand. If someone with such a traumatic life can achieve it, then anyone can. The flaw is that our yoni holds all our negative emotions. It holds the emotional pain of being ridiculed as a child. It holds the heartbreak of a young love. It holds the pain of losing a child. It holds the trauma of rape. It holds the trauma of child abuse. It holds the emotional pain from your childhood all the way to your adult life. It basically holds any emotional pain from your past. This pain is trapped deep within the walls of your yoni.

Your body holds all of these pains inside your yoni tissues and reproductive organs. For some special people. I call them special because they overcame hardships that many of us can never fathom. They overcame things that no human should endure. They survived an unimaginable and unthinkable pain many of us don't understand. It holds the pain of that intense emotional and physical abuse. Of course, you can imagine this one; it holds the pain of sexual abuse. Any kind of trauma is held in this sacred place. It is held there to protect you and keep you aware. It is meant to protect you in some way by creating symptoms that make you aware. But feeling that physical pain doesn't make you aware of anything unless you reached a flowing state.

Granted, if you suffered abuse or trauma, there might be some additional treatments that will enable you to release that trapped emotional energy from the depths of those tissues. That can be achieved with a special treatment called Yoni massage, which I experienced with Michelle Alva, a close friend. This unique massage targets the pelvic floor muscles and vaginal tissues to reduce tension, pain, emotions, and trauma from the past. I can tell you from personal experience it is a beautiful experience that brings tears to your eyes and awakens you from your slumber. I am not a pelvic floor physical therapist or a yoni massage specialist. That isn't the point here. I'm simply letting you know that if you had any emotional or physical pain or trauma in your past, you might need a little additional help to release it from your Yoni. You can get that help from a licensed therapist that has experience in this unique massage. I personally loved the experience with Michelle. Now that you understand that you hold stress and inflammation there, how do you get rid of stress there? What can you do every day to calm your body? What can you do to tap into the healing capabilities of your body? That is easy: Kegel.

The final key steps are Kegel exercises to release stress, tension, emotions, and anxiety from your yoni. Squeeze your pelvic floor muscles by squeezing the muscles between your anus and your vagina. If you aren't sure you are squeezing properly, a pelvic floor physical therapist can help you. But a simple trick is to place your hands where your pelvic bone ends, and your tummy begins. If you have a C-section scar like me, that is the exact spot to place your hand over. As you squeeze the pelvic floor muscles, you will feel in that spot. I know no one does this enough. But the truth is, your vagina is a muscle, and it needs to be exercised regularly. To maintain muscle tone, it is essential. But that is a huge part of all reproductive issues. This enhances blood flow and builds muscles.

My muscles are so strong that I void quickly, and it

surprises people. The stream is strong and quick. The fluid is lymphatic and urinary fluid. This is only possible because I built up those muscles that many of us let go. If you let go, there are a ton of issues that can develop if you don't use those muscles. The amazing part is that using this routine enhances brain function, calms your senses, sooths your nervous system, and improves your pelvic health. Get to your Kegels. Your body deserves it.

You can use it in the morning to energize and calm down; in the evening to relax, release, and let go. Another great tool to use to build up these essential muscles is a Yoni egg. It is a little egg made from crystals that you insert into your vagina to strengthen the muscles. There are different sizes, and you can choose the one that is most comfortable for you. You can start slow, using it for a few hours, and then increase its use. I am so accustomed to it that I can leave it all day. This also helps with dryness and lubrication issues, because it enhances blood flow easily and effortlessly to your pelvis. I am so comfortable with the egg that I can wear it all day. It helps improve your bladder control, urine stream, lubrication, orgasms, muscle tone, and so much more. I choose crystals because they are made from the earth. I tried artificial ones made from other ingredients, and they simply feel foreign and often cause other sensitivities or issues. Our bodies deserve the most natural ingredients, and crystals provide all the benefits. Now, it's time to learn how to bring everything together and enhance pelvic flow.

Enhancing Yoni Flow

Now, let's get back to your yoni and ways to get your energy flowing again. This process is a simple routine to reduce the tension and inflammation in your yoni. This will enable you to flow the energy easily through your body, reducing your hormonal fluctuations and physical pain. The fun thing I learned is that it helped stretch my fascia, thus reducing symptoms of IBS, too. The first thing I teach in my course is this simple breathing and stretch routine that I call "dragonfly." Place your hands behind your neck and relax. Place the soles of your feet together and open your knees wide apart. The position looks like the wings of a dragonfly.

It's a position that opens up your pelvic floor muscles and abdomen to help you relax. It helps reduce the stress response in your body by calming your nervous system. You know this as the fight or flight response. Many of us are stuck in a chronic state of stress because this response doesn't stop. The dragonfly breath technique helps calms the nervous system. It taps into self-healing and self-calming potential. Using this routine several times a day enhances its effectiveness. It is a great way to get energized in the morning and calm your senses. Have you ever woken up worrying about something or feeling anxious? This little position will help you relax, and it's super simple. It is also an amazing way to calm and relax before bed. The best part is that it's easy. If you can't get in the exact position because of mobility issues, you can make an X instead. Simply lay flat and extend your arms and feet out like an X.

Then, while in this position, you use the five-five-five breath that I taught you before. With each exhale, you open your mouth and let out a moan. The moan can be any sound that comes up, but some examples are, "ahh," "ehh," "ohh," "lalala." This funny sound helps relax your throat and pelvic floor simultaneously. I enjoy inventing new ones or alternating between a few. It doesn't really matter. The point is that you use your vocals to release the emotions and feelings from your body. You use your vocals to express yourself. Just breath, relax, and let go. Now, it's time to use your Kegel exercise. Gently squeeze the muscles between your vagina and anus. Now, combine it all together. As you squeeze those muscles, breath in using the five-five-five breath; and as you let go, relax the muscles again. This is amazing for brain and yoni fitness. Using this routine for five to ten minutes twice a day is a spectacular way to reduce stress and inflammation in your body. If you have a yoni egg, insert it prior to the activity and strengthen those muscles more efficiently when you combine it with this routine.

Climactic Stretch

I also developed a routine called climactic stretch, which progressively relaxes the muscle tension throughout your body by targeting your unique tension areas. The fun thing I learned is that it also improves lymphatic flow and reduces inflammation. I have a chronic debilitating condition called EDS III, which impacts connective tissues, muscles, and all organs. This routine helped me overcome those tight muscles, tender sore spots, and numb and tingly areas; it even improved bruising. Most people with my condition chronically become debilitated as the muscles shrink, shrivel, and lose circulation. Yet, I overcame carpel tunnel, pyriformis syndrome, bursitis, plantar fasciitis, etc. All of these pesky diagnoses deal with tight connective tissues and inflammation.

It is a slow, gentle, progressive stretch that elongates and lengthens your muscles. It improves mobility, motion, and circulation. I know this because half my body was impaired and numb for twenty years. I had lack of function in my right hand and carpel tunnel. Opening doors and bottles was almost impossible with my right hand. I still get stuck in occasional doors with those round handles. It makes me laugh every time. But I know I made huge accomplishments in my physical state because of this loving routine. I've worked up to getting rid of the splints and supportive devices I used to use every day. What's this routine? How do I do it? I'll explain a simple routine in the next section, but the basic principle begins with a stretch routine for any muscle in your body.

You can find a ton of stretches on YouTube if you aren't sure. Or, check out my channel and see my routine. The best way to learn my crazy, silly movements is in a class with me, but I will give you an idea. Have you ever stretched your quad? Stand up and support yourself. Now, bend your right knee and grab your right foot with your right hand. Perfect. Now is the tricky and fun part. As you balance and support yourself in this stretch routine, squeeze your pelvic floor muscles. Yep, the big secret to this routine is Kegel exercise. It promotes lymphatic drainage using stretching, breathing, and Kegel exercises. The routine helps improve blood flow all over your body. It reduces inflammation and toxins. The Kegel exercise is the secret to brining it all together and making your body a stress fighting machine. I know it's super weird and awkward at first, but with practice it becomes easy. I will show you a super easy way to use this routine daily. If you use all these little strategies, you will be a Kegel master and stress-fighting machine.

Flowing through Climactic Stretch

It's hard to show you how to stretch in a book. Using the visual images I showed you before, I will guide you to do a simple climactic stretch for your Yoni. Get into the dragonfly or X position on your bed or couch. Lay back with a pillow supporting your neck and back. Get comfortable and begin breathing. Use the five-five-five breath and relax. You might feel stiff and tight the first few times, because you never tried this before. Your inner thighs are connected with your yoni and they hold that emotional pain, too. The goal here is to get the energy flowing from your pelvis down your legs.

Now that you are comfortable in the dragonfly position and you went through the breathing routine, you should feel a little more relaxed. Now, with the soles of your feet together, hold in your core and wiggle your hips from side to side. It is a gentle side-to-side motion, moving those tense tight inner thigh muscles to loosen them up. While you wiggle, it's time to Kegel. Perfect. Exactly like that. Keep wiggling for a count of twenty.

Now, take a moment to feel your body. Do you still feel tight? Are you tighter on the left? Are you tighter on the right? Focus on that side where you are tight. Now, gently push your knee down into the couch, flexing that thigh a little deeper. Breath in and out using the five-five-five breath and let out that moan. If you are extra tight repeat it a few times until you feel more relaxed and open. Now, do it on the other side, too. It might not be as tight but the goal here is to flow evenly. That was pretty simple right. You can totally do that twice a day in your bed or couch. You can do it outside on a yoga mat, too, but I find it is easier on a soft cushion to stretch the inner thighs more efficiently and gently.

Energy Flowing State

Now, to keep our energy flowing during the day is not so easy. You can't just bust out into a dragonfly position at work, in your car, or at a party. But there are simple strategies you can use to inconspicuously enhance the flow of energy in your body. By now, you know your body is filled with energy, and it's impacted by the emotional and physical energies around us. It is impacted by stressful situations and events. It is affected by confrontational conversations and people. These obstacles and challenges can happen anytime and anywhere. Learning these little hacks will help calm and relax you in any of these situations.

The most important thing to remember is that you will be combining these simple tools with your breathing technique. I know that if you are in a public place, you aren't going to want to make the "ahh" sound, but you can exhale out your mouth and use your imagination to allow you to feel like you are. Yep, totally weird. I get it. This crazy lady is telling me to breath and imagine I am making an "ahh" sound. I'm doing this because your mind is powerful, and your imagination is, too. Even though you aren't able to actually do it, the simple imagination helps you connect with that calm much more effectively. Here are some positions you can use to relax using the principles of energy medicine. It will help reconnect the left side of your body to the right side of your body. It will help release those negative feelings and emotions. You can feel a change within a few minutes. But again, combining it with breathing and imagery is ten times more powerful than just using the position alone. I also teach some more advanced strategies that combine the routine with hypnosis for an expedited transformation, but I can't explain that here. Here is the first position:

Self-Love Hug: It's time for a little self-love and affection with a hug. Simply cross your arms and grab your shoulders with the opposite hand. Your right hand is on your left shoulder and your left hand is on your right shoulder. If you feel tension or tightness, take a few moments to massage and caress those tender spots. If you don't, simply hold that position while you complete the five-five-five breath. Of course, Kegel while your breath. Squeeze your pelvic floor as you inhale and hold. On your exhale, release those muscles

Pregnant-Princess: Yep, crazy name, but that is what I see when I do it, so here it is. I call it pregnant princess because when you are pregnant, you rub your belly. It's weird, but fun. Place your right hand on your forehead like a crown. y, your left hand on your pelvis or lower abdomen. If you have any tension, take a moment to rub the area in a circular motion. Now, hold the position while you practice the five-five-five breath. Remember to Kegel as you inhale and let go as you exhale. Continue to rub your belly or simply keep your hand on your belly. Skin-to- skin contact is the most effective, so lift up that shirt. It's a great technique when you feel stressed, and you can do it in your chair or even on the toilet. Lol. Yes, I said toilet. You are feeling tired or stressed. Maybe your mind isn't flowing, or you are stuck on a project unable to think. Maybe you have brain fog. Let's add a little extra step here. As you breathe in, deeply roll your eyes upward. Yep, it feels weird. Your eyes roll up into your eyebrows as you breathe. Each time you inhale, do this. It gets the energy flowing into your brain again and enhances focus. How do you feel?

Criss-Cross Hug: Extend your arms in front of you, palms facing outward. Extend your right arm over your left or vice versa – whatever is comfortable for you. It feels awkward at first. Now, interlock your fingers together. n. Now, rotate your arms while interlocked and bring your hands into your chest. Your hands should be resting on your chest near your heart. Now, practice the five-five-five breath. Of course, as you breathe, squeeze those pelvic floor muscles. Alright, so there they are – a few simple strategies that you can use anytime and anywhere. Don't worry about the people around you. If they ask, you can tell them. They are probably are just curious to know what you are doing. By now, you understand the benefit of creating a supportive routine for yourself. You know that you can use some simple strategies during the day to calm you. You are ready to move on to the next chapter.

Yoni Unleashed

Missy was grateful for her transformation. She finally enjoyed amazing sex with her new boyfriend. She worked hard on her transformation and combined my program with yoni massage. She was amazed at how much trapped pain and trauma her rape left behind. Her favorite part of the routine is climactic stretch. She didn't realize her orgasmic potential until she began using this regularly. She was grateful that sex was no longer a painful and stressful experience. She was thankful that she could enjoy sex with her boyfriend. She finally was living the life she deserved, free of symptoms and pain. It all started with unveiling the truth of her trauma from the root.

CHAPTER 11: EVOLVE – SELF-LOVE AND REFLECTION

Self-Love Evolution

Elizabeth was, by far, my favorite story. She had no self-esteem, even though she was gorgeous. She was sexually abused as a child and told she was ugly and fat. The emotional and physical trauma left her feeling trapped inside her body. She was plagued with symptoms: chronic pain, debilitating symptoms, severe digestive issues, and chronic vaginal infections. She miraculously transformed her life and her health and found her freedom. Soon, I will unveil her transformation, but first, it's time to talk about your physical and emotional freedom.

Physical and Emotional Freedom

Freedom from illness and disease comes with the decision for change and a new lifestyle choice. It seems like wellness is an intricate process, but it's actually easy once you put it all into action. It's simply adding one new thing at a time until you have a routine that makes you thrive and flourish. The path to reducing symptoms within your body doesn't have to be complicated. It does, however, require awareness and action. By now, you are aware that there are many ways to impact the stress inside your body. You understand the physical and emotional root of your anxiety, pain, and symptoms. You practiced different strategies to create a sense of calm within you to impact both the emotional and physical root. It is clear now that your wellness is in your hands.

You know by now that no one can do this for you. The decision to change your health and your life is yours and yours alone. Reading this book was the first step in your transformation. Like how a caterpillar works hard to emerge and transform, you need to take action and work for what you dream. This is the chapter that puts it all together to show you it can be easy. Just like the caterpillar, you are evolving and changing. You were working on yourself, and it feels good.

Now it's just time to streamline the process and figure out your unique action plan. Your awareness keeps you connected with your body and lets you know exactly what, when, and how to respond. This awareness is your friend and will support you in your transformation. It is your signal of physical and emotional stress. It's also a beautiful sign and a gift once you are ready to see it. When you are aware and take action, everything suddenly falls into place, and you feel good. These happy feelings and good sensations make you want to keep moving forward. The new free-flowing hormones empower you to move towards your transformation. You understand now that transformation is a process of evolution and change.

THE TRUTH ABOUT IBS AND ANXIETY

You already began to support yourself through stressful situations. You know that when triggers happen, taking action makes you a stress-fighting machine. You know that ignoring this awareness only activates the nervous system, creating a buildup of stress throughout your body. You know that this ignorant state no longer serves the purpose and path you chose. You are ready and willing to shift your life and shift the way you feel. The ultimate goal is to live a life free of bloating, cramping, indigestion, pain, and anxiety. The goal is achieved by staying in tune with your awareness and taking action. I bet you think I'm a little crazy. You are thinking, "It is impossible to put all of these things into motion. I don't have time for all this stuff. It's too hard. It's too complicated. It's impossible." I heard all the stories. I even said them to myself. But when you realize that your goal is set and your plan is in motion, nothing is impossible. When you realize that your health, happiness, and joy depend on a little self-care and self-love, you will do it. I understand that some days are harder.

I understand that some days will be too complicated for everything. But the secret is that if you do these things several times a week, and have a few days where you focus more, your body will appreciate it. Even three days a week of more consistency is better than none. A couple days with a morning and bedtime routine works better than one. It's about you finding a balance and internal support system for yourself. It's about starting slow and adding in gradually. Dealing with the pain and constant symptoms isn't easy. I bet you are sick of it by now.

I know I was fed up with feeling like a whale inside my body. I was sick of looking pregnant and bloated at parties. I was sick of being trapped in my room for hours or days. When I decided my health, happiness, and joy were more important, everything shifted. I bet you are sick of being sick and tired. You are sick of it all. Using your awareness to take action is a super powerful gift. By now, you already know your triggers. You are well aware of your challenges and obstacles. You know what people upset you simply by being in the room. You know what people drain your energy. You know what it feels like inside your body when you are anxious or stressed. You know what it feels like when a muscle suddenly tightens during an uncomfortable conversation. Now, the job is yours. The task is waiting for you. Your body is sending you the message. Your body gave you a gift. It's the gift of awareness. The only thing your body wants back is a little self-loving attention.

What are you waiting for? What is holding you back? Are you ready to take the leap with me? So, let's do this. Let's plan a day of self-love and self-care. Let's get an idea of a day where everything falls into place and you kick ass at self-love. Let's also plan a day when the world seems to be throwing you curveballs every second and you need a quick relaxation. Let's plan a day where you have no time to take breaks, but you remember your morning and evening routine. Does that sound easier? Do you think you can handle that? Do you deserve to feel healthy? Do you deserve to feel better? I say absolutely, yes. You deserve to feel vibrant, healthy, and alive. You deserve to thrive. Let's go for it. Let's put it all together so you can see it is easy and effortless.

Evolution Unleashed

Before you get to the routine that will transform your life, let me explain Elizabeth's evolution. She was traumatized by her childhood experiences but worked hard on her transformation. She truly enjoyed her self-love routines and raved about how they made her feel. She listened to her hypnosis every day and created affirmation art to share with others. She evolved and began to see her beauty. She realized that she was hiding behind shades her whole life. She finally saw her beautiful pale skin, blue eyes, and black hair with new eyes. When she finally loved herself, something miraculous happened. She found true love. It was in her face the entire time, but she was too blind to see it. She was grateful and thankful for her newfound life and love. Now that you understand the true potential of self-love and appreciation, take a look at these easy routines that can transform your life as you evolve and change.

The Effortless Routines

Self-Love Ecstasy

The day you give it 100%, you are kicking ass and feeling fabulous because everything is falling into place. You are doing it all. You are a rock star. You do your morning mantra with quick stretch routine and dragonfly position before you get up. Use the five-five-five breath while in sacred surrender and moan when you exhale. Use "ahh" or any other sound. Use your Kegel exercises. Stretch a little while you brush your teeth with an affirmation repeating in your head. Try it with a five-five-five breath and a few Kegels, too. Driving to work, you listen to your favorite relaxing song or meditation. As you drive, you take in deep breaths and blow out the air in an "ahh" sound. Easy so far, right? No big deal – you got this. Then, you sing along to some fun and invigorating music. When the singer gets into vocals, you do it too. Any sound – just let it out. If something comes up and you want to scream, do it. No one is listening.

Morning meditation: You go outside into nature, feel the sun on your skin, pop in your earbuds, close your eyes, and listen to a guided meditation for fifteen to twenty minutes. Lay in dragonfly position. Do the five-five-five breath and Kegels. You feel energized and pumped to be super productive. Lunch Meditation: You eat your lunch and chat for a bit with a friend. Then, you pop in your earbuds and listen to a hypnotic intensive filled with affirmations for twenty minutes. You sit in any position. Do the five-five-five breath and a few Kegels. Afternoon workout: You go to the gym, play a sport, or do your favorite activity. You end it with breathing and stretches and release. You pop in your earbuds and listen to a meditation or hypnotic intensive. While you stretch those really sore areas, you breathe deeply using the five-five-five breath. Release any emotions that come up in that tender spot. A few extra Kegels make you a stress-fighting machine. You feel your muscles relaxing and loosening after that workout.

Massage: Today is an extra special day. You have an extra hour, and the massage therapist called you. It could be acupuncture, reiki, an Epson salt soak, a sensory deprivation tank, or any other alternative treatment you like. Today, you get an extra-special luxury just for you. If you pop in your earbuds, you can make it even more relaxing. Listen to ambient sounds, meditation, or a hypnotic intensive. Bring in your senses for an exponentially better relaxation benefit.

Car release: You drive home and sing along to the music. When they get into vocals, you just do it. Make those noises. Use your voice. If any emotions come up, let them out in a scream. Some songs may trigger memories or emotions. Let them go. You feel amazing, because today was a rock star day.

Journaling and creativity: Today was an awesome day. Nothing really challenging happened, but you want to journal. You write a journal about your day. Focus on giving gratitude and thanks to everything in your life. Give thanks for everything amazing that happened today. Appreciate all the beautiful things in your life. You use some color pencils to draw a border around your journal. It was such an amazing day.

TV stretch: You use your stretch-and-release routine while you watch TV. The most important position now is modified dragonfly (arms resting on your side). Just lay in this position and focus on stretching your inner thighs. If any negative emotions come up when you watch TV, you release them in the moment. Raise your left arm into the air and feel the relaxation deepen. Take in a deep five-five-five breath and say in your head: "I release any worry, shame, guilt, or fear from my body. I am free to live a happy and joyful life. I am free." You notice that your sore, tight muscles are relaxing and soon you will be ready for sleep (or sex – whichever comes first. Lol.)

Bedtime routine: Get into dragonfly and do a five-five-five breath. Kegel a few more times. Moan and groan as you exhale. Caress your body in an upwards motion. Feel the calm and peaceful feeling throughout your body. That's right. The caresses are soothing and comforting. If you are in the mood, have sex. It's perfectly natural. If you are exhausted, then drift off to sleep.

Orgasmic release: If you choose sex, it's completely up to you, but the release is a great way to calm the body for a deep, restful night's sleep. I usually have sex every night. I usually sleep even deeper when I do. Okay, this is the fun part. Your partner might think you are weird at first. When you feel a climax, use the new sounds you learned: "ahh," "ohh," "lalala," "ehh." Watch your body release everything completely, leaving you filled with happy hormones. Use your Kegels. Ladies, I guarantee your partner will like when you use this technique.

That was just a kick-ass day. You rocked it completely. You did it all and then some. Your body loved it. Your mind appreciated it. It just gave you an edge for the rest of the week. You felt amazing the entire day and you slept like a baby. Even if you get most of these things done three days a week, you are a rock star at self-love.

Self-Love on a Rainy Day

This is literally a day that makes you want to cry, because so much crap is falling on your lap. You want to scream. There isn't much time to relax and unwind, but a few strategic ideas will help you tackle the stress anyway.

Morning mantra with quick stretch routine in firefly position before you get up. Use the five-five-five breath and Kegels. Moan when you exhale – "ahh" or any other sound. A little stretch while you brush your teeth with an affirmation repeating in your head. A few Kegels wouldn't hurt.

Car release: Driving to work, you listen to your favorite relaxing song or meditation. As you drive, you take in deep breaths using the five-five-five breath. Blow out the air in an "ahh" sound. Easy so far, right? No big deal – you got this. At the traffic light, you do a few Kegels while you breathe deeply.

Morning meditation: You go outside into nature, feel the sun on your skin, pop in your earbuds, close your eyes, and listen to a guided meditation for fifteen to twenty minutes. You can get in any position and use the five-five-five breath. As you exhale, you say, "Ohh." If you get into firefly, it is amazing. All you need is a yoga mat. No matter what, don't skip this step. It might seem like you want to. It might seem impossible, but do it, even if it's only ten minutes. Don't give up on yourself. You deserve better, and this will help you.

Quick breath release: You just got a phone call that makes you want to scream; a new deadline you need to complete ASAP. It seems like the day is getting worse by the moment. Maybe you have a knot somewhere in your body now. It's time to breath. You can stretch at your desk. No one needs to know what you are doing. No one is watching. If they are, go to the bathroom. Use the five-five-five breath and exhale with an "ohh" sound. As you stretch, say in your head or out loud, "I release this stress from my body. I am calm, peaceful, and serene. Everything will happen easily and effortlessly. I got this." It was five minutes, and wow you feel better. Jump back into work and get it done.

Bathroom break: You only had time for three bathroom breaks today. But you took your time wisely. As you walked to the bathroom, you did your five-five-five breath. When you got inside, you did a little stretch and release. You focus on your arms and legs the most. It was a long day. It's time to get those muscles moving. You breathe and release. It was a brief break, but you feel amazing. Get back to work.

Lunch: At your desk. You pop in your earbuds and listen to a meditation or hypnotic intensive. You don't have to close your eyes. Just listen. Eat your food calmly. Chew and swallow slowly. You might only have ten minutes but relax and enjoy them. If you are able to keep the earbud in one ear while you work do it. Listen to another hypnotic intensive, ambient noise, or meditation while you finish that task. You got this.

Afternoon workout: You go to the gym and play a sport or your favorite activity. You end it with breathing and stretching and release. You pop in your earbuds and listen to a meditation or hypnotic intensive. While you stretch those really sore areas, you breathe deeply using the five-five-five breath. Release any emotions that come up in that spot. You feel your muscles relaxing and loosening easily after that workout.

Car release: The day rushed by, and you have tons of errands to run. You sing along to your favorite dance songs. Get into it and wiggle in your seat at the stop light. Dance when the car is stopped. Sing at the top of your lungs. Scream if you want to. As you drive, you take in deep breaths and blow out the air on an "ahh" sound. This is fun. You might be running around, but the singing distracted you from the crazy afternoon. You feel awesome.

Bedtime routine: Don't ever miss this step. Today was hard enough. You deserve a little self-love time. Get into sacred surrender and do a five-five-five breath. Moan and groan as you exhale. Kegel a few times while you breathe. Caress your body in an upwards motion. Feel the calm and peaceful feeling throughout your body. That's right. The caresses are soothing and comforting. If you are in the mood, have sex; if not, just close your eyes and drift off to sleep.

Orgasmic release: It was a rough day, and you really want to relax. This is an amazing way to let everything go. You might need a little toy, wine, or massage beforehand, but get in motion. Your deep, restful night's sleep is just a few orgasms away. I usually have sex every night. If I don't, the sleep is not so restful. Okay, this is the fun part. When you feel a climax, use the Kegels and the new sounds you learned: "ahh," "ohh," "lalala," "ehh." Watch your body release everything completely, leaving you filled with happy healthy hormones. You will sleep like a baby.

Self-Love on a Bumpy Day

Today is showing you no mercy. You have too many deadlines, and things keep happening. The only time you have is a quick bite to eat and a bathroom break. Perfect, not a problem. You can do this. You got this. You started off your day right with your morning mantra and a quick stretch routine in firefly before you get up. Use the five-five-five breath. Kegel and moan when you exhale – "ahh" or any other sound. A little stretch while you brush your teeth with an affirmation repeating in your head. A couple Kegels for an extra bonus.

Car release: Driving to work, you listen to your favorite relaxing song or meditation. As you drive, you take in deep breaths (five-five-five) and blow out the air in an "ahh" sound. Easy so far, right? No big deal – you got this.

Morning meditation: You go outside into nature, feel the sun on your skin, pop in your earbuds, close your eyes, and listen to a guided meditation for fifteen to twenty minutes. No matter what, don't skip this step. It might seem like you want to. It might seem impossible, but do it, even if it's only ten minutes. Don't give up on yourself. You deserve better, and this will help you. If you have a yoga mat, get into firefly. If not, get into any position. Do a little stretch and Kegel.

Quick breath release: You just got a phone call that makes you want to cry; a new task needs to be completed ASAP. It seems like the day is getting worse by the moment. Maybe you have a knot somewhere in your body now. It's time to breath. No one needs to know what you are doing. No one is watching. You stretch a few minutes in your chair. You use the five-five-five breath. As you exhale, say, "I release this stress from my body. I am calm, peaceful, and serene. Everything will happen easily and effortlessly. I got this." It was five minutes, and wow you feel better. Jump back into work and get it done. You can do it.

Bathroom break: You only had time for a few bathroom breaks today. But you took your time wisely. As you walked to the bathroom, you did your five-five-five breath and Kegel. When you get inside, you do a little stretch and release. You focus on your arms and legs the most. Move those muscles and breath. It was a brief break, but you feel amazing. Get back to work.

Car release: The day rushed by, and you have tons of things do to. You want to go to the gym, but time is slim. Let's get silly with it. Sing along to your favorite workout music. Get into it and wiggle, jiggle, and move at the stop light. At the traffic light, squeeze your abdominal muscles and do Kegels. Keep singing at the top of your lungs. Use that voice, baby. You got this. As you drive, you take in deep breaths and blow out the air in an "ahh" sound at least five times.

Journaling and creativity: Today was a rough day. There is a lot to get off your chest. Many emotions came up. It's time to vent. Take a few minutes to get it out. Write in a journal or type it into your computer, but get it out of your mind. For an added bonus, grab a coloring page and get creative. Draw something. Color something. It doesn't matter what it looks like. Just do it.

Bedtime routine: Don't miss this step. Today was hard enough. You deserve a little self-love and relaxation. This is easy and only takes a few minutes. Get into firefly and do a five-five-five breath. Moan and groan as you exhale. Caress your body in an upwards motion. Kegel a few times while you breathe. Feel the calm and peaceful sensations rushing throughout your body. That's right. Gentle sensations are soothing and comforting. Sex is always an option. If you are tired, go to sleep.

Orgasmic release: It was a rough day and you really want to get to sleep, but your mind isn't shutting off. This is an amazing way to let everything go. Read something sexy. You might need a little toy, wine, or massage beforehand, but get in motion. Your deep, restful night's sleep is just a few orgasms away. Don't forget to use your sexy sounds. When you feel a climax, say, "ahh," "ohh," "lalala," "ehh," Let those happy hormones flow. Squeeze those pelvic muscles. Release that sacred sensual energy. Now, it's time to drift off to sleep, you rockstar.

I know it seems like a lot of work. You are thinking it will take too much time and effort. But it actually will make you more productive and efficient in everything else you do. You are just changing the way you do things a little to make it more beneficial and nurturing to your body. Once you get in the routine, the process will be easy and effortless. You will be surprised at all the other things you will accomplish when you feel relaxed, calm, and focused.

CHAPTER 12: BURY THE PAST – SUPPORT AND ACCOUNTABILITY FOR SUCCESS

Getting Accountable

It's time to bury the past and move on to a beautiful future. This is the moment you shift and transform. Trust me, I understand. It seems impossible. It seems unrealistic. There might even be words popping into your head. "I can't do this. I'm too busy. This is too hard." I understand your hesitation. I understand the emotional and physical struggle it entails. It's hard to develop accountability and support when you are the only one invested in your transformation. Sure, you can find friends that support you and express their pride in your accomplishments. But how long will that really last?

You might be able to get a friend to join you in your transformational journey. You may even make huge leaps on your own. But the simple fact is that I wish I found a coach, doctor, or mentor to smooth my path seven years ago. I wish that I had someone to direct and guide me through the obstacles and challenges. I wish I tackled these health challenges faster. I wish I was more autonomous and dedicated to my self-love from the beginning. I wish I had a shoulder to cry on. I wish I connected with someone who lived my pain. I wish I found someone who experienced the struggle I was going through. I wish that my journey was easier and faster.

Most of all, I wish that for you. My hope is that you evolve and change easily and effortlessly using this technique. In pure honesty, if I was in your shoes right now and I found someone that truly understood my unique pain, I would say, "Of course, yes, sign me up." But I wasn't that lucky – it was meant for me to struggle, fail, persevere, and push through. It was important for me to hit rock bottom and deal with my challenges alone. My pain and hardships brought me to this moment. It brought me to the point where I can use my pain to propel others forward. My pain opened my eyes to my unique gifts. It empowered me to find my way out of illness and disease. It empowered me to inspire others to find their unique wellness.

I know my pain and struggle gives others hope for a better life. That is why I believe that if you truly want to change now, if you truly want to tackle your symptoms now, then get support in the process. Find a friend, colleague, or mentor that connects with you on a deeper level. It has to be someone that experienced the struggles you face. It has to be someone that is willing to get down in the dirt with you. The best support for you will be someone that evolved and emerged from rock bottom. Why? Because that is the person that understands your deepest and darkest moments. That is the person that can motivate you. That is the person that can keep you on track. That person will help you put your obstacles and challenges into perspective. That person can give you strategies to tackle your stress in the moment. That person has a unique gift because they lived your pain and transformed themselves. That special gift is here for you to accept and receive with grace and gratitude.

Support Helps You Thrive

Do you still doubt the importance of a support system? Here is why my journey was so long, traitorous, and tedious. The subconscious obstacles in your mind are super powerful. These engrained beliefs were inside you since childhood. These pesky things create a sense of doubt within you that is practically impossible to tackle alone. I tried a bunch of times and failed over and over again. Until I started working with coaches, mentors, and colleagues. Yes, I worked with many. Nothing shifted for me without support. I kept falling down, falling apart, and picking up the pieces slowly. I worked with four to five coaches and mentors over the past year as I evolved and learned new things. This past year was really when the true transformation happened. Thanks to my support system I was able to shift and sustain changes.

If I didn't have a helping hand during the really hard times, I would stay stuck once again at rock bottom. Being stuck sucks. It means it takes you months or years to get up and move forward. It means that all the progress you made goes down the drain over and over. It can take you years to reach that success point, rather than months. It means you start all over an infinite amount of times until you finally make it. My subconscious mind took me more than a year to tackle. I used live coaches, recorded programs, mindfulness applications, mentoring sessions, support groups, and online programs. I used pre-recorded hypnosis, face-to-face hypnosis, and many other programs and tools over the past few months. I tackled them quickly, because I had a ton of valuable resources and tools at my disposal. Trust me, I tried all the online free stuff on YouTube, free webinars, free courses – free wasn't working for my brain.

My brain is just like your brain: it needs to make an investment. If you want to achieve anything, you need to be all in. You need to make a decision to invest in your personal development, and free doesn't allow you to do that. For your brain to *invest,* you need to make a conscious decision to *invest* in your personal growth and development. I wish that I figured that out seven years ago. It actually cost me much more time and money to go at it alone. I wish I found a support system early on that knew exactly how to help and guide me.

Your journey doesn't have to be that difficult, but a support system is crucial. There are many obstacles in your path to a healthy lifestyle. In today's society, food, drinks, and self-gratification are publicized and beautified everywhere. Everyone wants to eat the next trendy meal. Everyone wants to have that delectable desert. Everyone wants to indulge their inner emotional demons with food or drink. Everyone is struggling with overcoming their addictions. Everyone has a vice to overcome. The fact is that the media, television, and movies keep throwing more at you. When things are in your face, it makes it ten times harder to accomplish your goals.

You will see challenges in many different situations, events, and life experiences. You will be enticed by television shows, commercials, and movies. You will be pulled in by coupons and deals. You will be pushed by friends to try things you desperately want to avoid. You will be ridiculed for trying to eat healthy. You will be made fun of for being different. You will face a ton of hard times in a path to your wellness. For those reasons, you need a friend, supporter, and confidant. Find someone that gives you valuable feedback, resources, and tools to tackle the emotional and physical obstacles in your path. Your support system will help you thrive and pick up the pieces.

Your support system can and will smooth your way and make the path to evolution easier. The cost of trying to tackle food, drink, and addictions on your own is exponentially difficult. Though your deepest desire is to stay on track, temptation can throw you off. The cost is severe, with debilitating symptoms and pain. It will impact your health, happiness, finances, social life, etc. It will bring back those symptoms you were trying desperately to avoid.

Lack of support will throw you right back into the life you are trying to avoid. It will mean you will spend more time in the hospital and doctors' offices for treatments you really don't want. It means more prescriptions to try and cover those symptoms. Then, new symptoms begin to emerge from the prescription that is supposed to help. It means that everything you worked for until this moment will be wiped away. You will need to start all over a bunch of times until you make it. If I tally up all my struggles over the past seven years – all those surgeries, all those prescriptions, all those injections, all those procedures, all those emergency room visits, and all those doctors' visits – the cost was over $500,000. That is being conservative, because I am sure it was much more. A hospital visit alone with admission costs more than $100,000.

I spent countless hours in emergency rooms. I spent a myriad of hours in doctor's appointments. I spent so much time looking for an alternative that I didn't see my path. I was blinded by the white suite and didn't realize I was not meant to be treated inside a box. My path to wellness had to be outside of the box. It had to be outside of the conventional medicine bubble. I had to remove the blinders that were holding me back. Staying stuck is the result of keeping those blinders on. Staying in limbo feels like your body is collapsing and the end is approaching. Staying in that pain sucks. Feeling like your body is being taken over by aliens stinks. Feeling like you can't enjoy life because your symptoms took over your body isn't worth it.

Those struggles and obstacles in your path are the exact reason a support system is essential. Finding a friend, colleague, or mentor that evolved and emerged from rock bottom will propel you forward. They picked up the pieces over and over again. They changed and transformed. Getting advice from someone who lived it is different than getting advice from a doctor that has no clue what you are experiencing. Getting advice and support from a friend that didn't overcome the obstacles you seek to prevail over isn't going to push you forward on a path to success.

If success is what you seek, then don't do it alone. Get the support you need. Find someone that connects with your heart and pulls those strings to help you evolve. If this book didn't make you feel your pain, then find another one that does. I know that the perfect person is out there for you. You just need to be open and ready to find your support system. The question is, are you ready to *invest* in your wellness? Are you ready to leave the past behind and *transform* your life? Are you ready to *thrive*? All those challenges and obstacles I wrote about so far are external. These are forms of external resistance to your progress. They provide you will temptation that can throw you off track. They entice you with the things you are trying to avoid. They make it so much harder to accomplish your goals. But the biggest demon in your way is yourself.

You are the biggest obstacle to overcome. Your resistance to change is the reason you will fail repeatedly. Your inner child wants to stay safe and stuck. Your inner child wants to stay hidden. Your inner child is scared and fearful of getting hurt. Your dreams will be crushed over and over again if you allow your internal and external resistance to win. It will test you and try you over and over again. Find your support system to help you *thrive* and reach your goals efficiently, effectively and make it seem effortless and easy. Trust me, you still have to work at it, but it will make the process is smoother for you. With their support and guidance, the evolution will be seamless and effortless. The accountability and support propel you forward.

The consistency and follow-ups improve your perseverance and resilience. The path toward your deepest desires and dreams for your life. Your body and your wellness are exponentially easier with a support system. After all, your ultimate goal is to overcome those pesky symptoms. You want to feel alive, vibrant, and free again. You want to feel like a younger, healthier version of yourself. You want to find that healthy version of yourself that is hiding deep within you. You want to feel sexy, energetic, happy, and vibrant. You want to have the freedom to live the life you dream of – free of bloating, constipation, diarrhea, heartburn, anxiety, and pain.

You want to stop those horrible symptoms that keep you locked in your house or sitting on the couch at a party. You want to live the life of your dreams and kick your IBS, symptoms, and anxiety to the curb. You want to toss those pesky negative emotions into the trash. You want to live and be free from all those physical and emotional hardships. Most of all, you want to succeed and be *free*. The secret to success is to believe and commit with a support system. Use this technique and get support through the process to achieve your dream. If you truly want to succeed, the choice is in your hands.

Do you want to propel yourself to the next level? Do you want to finally overcome those horrible IBS symptoms? Do you want to *thrive* in life even without anxiety? Do you want to remove pain and debilitating symptoms from your life? Do you want to tackle your obstacles and succeed? The decision is yours to make. It's time to find your support system. It's time to find someone that understands your pain. It's time to find someone that reached for the stars and overcome it all.

Your support system might be a friend, colleague, mentor, or coach. It doesn't matter who it is, as long as you get one. It might be me, and I hope it is. If you made it this far in the book, there is something about me that you are intrigues you. There is something connecting you to my pain. There is something you see in me that you want for yourself. If that is true, if that is your truth, it's time to decide. Do you want to *thrive*? Your success is only a free phone call away. You have nothing to lose and everything to gain. Are you worth it? I think you are. I think everyone is. Everyone deserves to feel vibrant, vivacious, and alive. Are your ready to *thrive*? Do you want to feel *Free to Fly*? Get a support system and do it. I believe in you.

CHAPTER 13: CONCLUSION: BECOME FREE FLOWING MACHINE

Free Flowing is Effortless

Are you a free-flowing machine? I hope you are on the path to becoming one. This book was a little piece of my passion and purpose in life. I wrote this book specifically for you. If you made it this far, it was definitely for you. You are powerful and resilient. You can overcome those obstacles and challenges. You can fight the internal and external resistance. Most of all, you can achieve everything you dream. The path to your emergence is in this book. You have most of the tools to go at it alone. You even have a willing and waiting support system if you want to jump all in and tackle it quickly. It is possible for you to reduce those symptoms of anxiety, cramping, bloating, indigestion, and pain. It is possible to make your body work the way it was designed and created. You can do it all and have it all. I gave you all the tools that helped my clients achieve success with love and support. Everything I shared in this special book comes from the bottom of my heart. I know that my difficult journey was my path, but it doesn't have to be yours. I hope you achieve your dreams much faster than I did. I hope you can transform the way you feel inside your body quickly, easily, and effortlessly. I hope that the obstacles and challenges don't stop you from achieving your goals. I send you blessings and love on this journey to find your unique wellness. I hope the path to your wellness becomes easy and effortless with these techniques.

My path wasn't easy, but it led me to creating the *Unleashed Technique*. This little method took me seven years of trials, tribulations, and pain to create. I bring it all to you with love. If I can help you transform your life easily and effortlessly in weeks or months rather than years, then my hardships weren't in vain. My pain and suffering were completely worth it if they help you. I hope you are able to apply these silly, creative, and fun things into your life and achieve your dreams. You are worth it. I know you deserve it. This method is my secret gift to you. It's the way I became a free-flowing machine. It's the way I thrive in my life. It is the way I left chronic illness, debilitating pain, IBS, and anxiety in the past. It is the way I push forward and become a better version of myself every day. I evolve and change every day into a better version of myself. Life is an evolution, and if you aren't evolving, you stay stuck. Let's recap my little silly and crazy strategies again. Let's recap the steps in the *Unleashed Technique*:

Undo the Root

By now, you understand the root cause of illness and disease. You understand your IBS and anxiety results from a combination of the two. I discussed the emotional and physical stress as the root causes of illness, disease, and symptoms. Conventional medicine doesn't really help you tackle the issue at the root because it simply covers things up symptoms with prescriptions. That's why my process is outside of the box – to create a true path to healing and repair. Tackling the physical root is established by creating a nutritional support system that fuels your body and makes it a super healing machine. It gives your body the nutrients, herbs, and nutrition it needs to flourish and thrive. This chapter also gave you resources to tackle symptoms during flare ups to take quick and effective action. This foundation helps give you the energy, stamina, and vitality to propel forward and tackle the emotional root. By now, you recognize that not all herbs and nutrients are created equal. You understand that those that are truly backed by scientific research are highly beneficial to the body's healing process. This chapter gave you the foundational support system to address the physical root. Now that you understand that essential component, the rest of this program will help address that making it seem easy and effortless.

Nurture the Body

Your body deserves to work efficiently and effectively to tackle the inflammation and the physical root of your symptoms. This chapter paves a way to identifying inflammatory foods and food sensitivities to help reduce the symptoms at hand. The chapter showed you how to *thrive* in life by eliminating inflammatory foods from your diet first. This helps your body *rest, recover, restore,* and *repair*. The short elimination phase is followed by a reintroduction phase. This enables you to develop a plan of action by slowly reintroducing foods into your diet. By increasing the variety of foods into your diet, you will slowly feel more satisfied and less deprived. But the most empowering part of this chapter is the realization that your body deserves better sources of fuel to propel you forward in your transformation. This creates a foundation for your body to heal and repair itself from the damage that was done in the past. This unique plan helps you tackle that pesky inflammation that keeps you stuck in bed with symptoms and pain. That nutritious fuel and supportive foundation paces the way to tackling your stress response to reduce the impact of the emotional root on your body.

Let Go of the Past

This chapter provides an easy foundation to build mindful practices for yourself. It provides a basic foundation to tackle the emotional root of your symptoms. It connects you with some simple techniques to understand the impact anxiety and stress have on IBS (bloating, indigestion, constipation, diarrhea, and pain). It connects you with the emotional root of your symptoms to truly begin your path to physical freedom from your symptoms. It focuses on reflecting on life's challenges to make mindful decisions for the future. It provides some simple breathing techniques to relax your mind and body. Now that you have some simple techniques, let's combine them with physical activities to release the stress from your tissues.

Energize and Release

Stress is an inevitable part of our daily lives. There is no way to stop the challenges and obstacles that will come your way. But there is a powerful way to impact your reaction to them. This is the most fun and transformational step in the process. Tackling the stress with physical and vocal release is the easiest way out of the stress response. Using your body as a powerful stress-releasing machine is easy and effortless once you know how to do it. Tapping into your voice and vocals helps tackle that emotional stress that is trapped inside you. You would be surprised how much stress you are holding in your throat and vocal cords. The issues in your tissues are caused by your emotional triggers and inflammation. Learning these fun and invigorating simple things will add a pep in your step. It empowers you to let go and brings you more joy and happiness. Now that you have a foundational stress release strategy, it's time to create healthier relationships for your future.

Affirm Your Success

Now that you have a kick-ass routine to tackle your stress, it's time to create healthier relationships using boundaries. Let's face it: you keep many feelings and emotions trapped inside. There are relationships that cause you more heartache and pain than the rest. There are people that drain your energy and make you feel inferior. There are many things that you allow in your life that aren't healthy for you. Your body sends you messages through pain and symptoms. That is why boundaries support you in the process. They protect you and keep you safe. This is integral part of changing the way you feel, because it establishes ground rules for your relationships. The most influential part of this chapter is affirmations for success. They empower you to transform those negative subconscious beliefs. These positive thoughts help engrain new positive beliefs in your mind that empower you to push through and evolve. Engraining these new healthy habits and beliefs into your subconscious mind paves the way for you to achieve your dreams. But the transformation of your subconscious is about to get a little deeper and more effective in the next chapter.

Succeed with Hypnosis

Our mind can make us or break us on the path to transformation. It can lead us on a path to success or stop us in our tracks. That is all because of those subconscious blocks from our past. These negative beliefs and emotions that were created in our minds long ago impact our behaviors and actions. Your subconscious beliefs are engrained from childhood experiences and impact us our entire lives. Meditations provide a brief and effective sense of calm and balance. It is easy to integrate into your daily routine to increase your intuition and resilience. Hypnosis is beneficial to transforming the subconscious blocks even more effectively by reframing the beliefs and engraining them in the subconscious mind. These two techniques will create a sense of *calm and serenity* in your day. Now we get to the most fun and relaxing part of the book to truly release the issues in your tissues.

Holistic Health

You are made up of energy, and it flows inside your body every day. But inflammation, stress, and illness cause the energy to get trapped inside the body. This happens when challenges and obstacles arise causing tension and symptoms in the body. The chapter explains some easy strategies to enhance the flow of energy in your body. This is truly when everything comes together to evolve your healing process. The flow of energy helps you tackle emotional and physical stress at its core. The best part of the process is yoni health, because it enhances blood flow to the pelvis, reducing symptoms in women. The fun benefit is the libido slowly returning, enhancing your orgasms and pleasure. This is the chapter that connects the dots in the journey to evolve and change your stress response. This chapter gave you a simple morning and evening routine to relax your nervous system and promote energy flow. You learned a few extra techniques to relax you and promote energy flow during the day.

Evolve

Now that you know all the steps in the *Unleashed Technique*, you will continue to evolve and grow. These self-loving practices keep you thriving and transforming. This is the chapter that brings everything together. It gives you easy daily routines to make the process simple and effortless. The more you use this process in your life, the more you evolve into the new version of yourself you seek. You evolve and change into a stress fighting machine that tackles obstacles and challenges in the moment. This awareness and action set you free from your debilitation symptoms. Are you ready to live your life and *thrive?*

The truth you realized by now is that your routine and choices in life pave the way for you to succeed or fail. You also know that *you* are the most important person in your life. That means you have to choose yourself sometimes to impact your life and the lives of those around you. This short chapter brings everything you learned together to make you a super stress-fighting machine. This is the chapter that makes all fun, silly, easy, and effortless. It places everything into perspective to give you a plan of action for your week. It empowers you to push through the hard days using awareness and action. It releases the chains that bind you to your pain by creating a self-loving routine that works for you. This unique routine will serve you on your path to evolution. This action plan is the key to unleashing your inner strength and thriving. This is where everything comes together that is easy to understand. It takes your life from stress to thriving by making self-love easy.

Dream

The last step is all yours. You are free to dream and live the life you deserve, because once you reach this step, you are a stress-fighting machine. You are a powerhouse and can achieve anything you put your mind and heart into. You own today. Go live it. Use your action and awareness to empower your evolution and transformation. It's time to become everything you dream, because your stress is no longer holding you back.

There you have it. Every last drop of knowledge I can possibly share in a tiny book. The secret to my success and my hope for you to achieve it, too. My dream is for you to achieve your dreams and live a life free of symptoms. The *Unleashed Technique* is the *easiest* and most efficient path to your evolution. I streamlined the process over seven years so that you could achieve it easily and effortlessly. It is a clean-cut way to get the result you need and desire. It is the *fastest* way to tackle those pesky symptoms that are holding you back. It is the way to free you from the anxiety, symptoms, and IBS that torture you in your current life. Everything is possible when you unleash your inner strength. Are you ready to *thrive*? Let's *thrive* in life together. I'm just a phone call away. It's time to evolve and change your future is waiting for you.

Acknowledgments

This book was a long time in the making. I actually started writing seven years ago at the beginning of my health journey. It was a path filled with obstacles and challenges, resulting in months and years where writing was not flowing. I always wanted to share my true feelings verbally, but writing was always easier for me. I was a poet in my childhood and teens, but my gifts went dormant for a long time. I thank my mom Diana for her interests in writing and poetry, because it always sparked my interest.

Writing brings me great joy and happiness. I enjoy writing in my journal, social media, blog, and newsletters for my tribe. I also enjoy writing fictional works that spark my creativity. Writing this book was definitely an intense process to complete, but the time flew so quickly. Honestly, I was shocked that I completed the manuscript in less than three weeks, especially considering I wrote most chapters early in the morning while everyone was asleep. I spent early mornings typing away before heading to work and still managed to finish quickly. I am so thankful that Angela Lauria popped into my Facebook feed in July. That amazing video finally got me off my ass to push me to writing the book I always dreamed. My subconscious tried to stop me from filling out the application by ensuring I had a few technology issues in the process, but I finally submitted, and the rest is history.

I was grateful and thankful when I joined the Author Incubator Program, because I was met with a vast community of like-minded individuals. The process was inspirational for me to create a meaningful book to reach more people. The support and accountability were amazing to keep me on track. They supported me through the difficult challenges and writing blocks that occurred along the way. I am thankful for Ramses Rodriguez for noticing I needed help even when I was too scared to ask. His guidance and support propelled me forward to achieve my dreams. To this day, I ask myself this powerful question when obstacles come in my way: "How are you going to mess this up?" That question reminds me that I am strong and resilient, regardless of the challenges that come my way.

Speaking of my path, I cannot express enough gratitude for Martha and Brooke. Their work literally changed the entire course of my life. Until I met them and studied their teachings, I had no idea that I had any amount of control over my thoughts, emotions, and my life. It was through them that I met Angela and was able to bring this book to fruition. Thank you, amazing women, for your work in the world and for showing up so courageously and authentically. You all are the example of what is possible.

I am grateful for Dr. Angel Veloso and Dr. Donato Arguelles. These two physicians actually showed me great love and support in my years of illness, pain, and disease. They cared for me with great compassion and love. Dr. Veloso was a guiding light that pushed me to a path of change as my body hit my health crisis. If he didn't open my eyes to my eminent death, I would not be here today.

To The Author Incubator team: Special thanks again to Dr. Angela Lauria, CEO and founder of The Author Incubator, for believing in me and my message. To my developmental editor, Mehrina Asif, and managing editor, Cory Hott; thanks for making the process seamless and easy. Many more thanks to everyone else at TAI, but especially Ramses Rodriguez for guiding me through my writing anxiety and helping me speak my truth.

To my former pediatric emergency team, I am so thankful for all of you that supported me during my health crisis. Many of us moved and travelled to different places, but you will always have a loving place in my heart.

To my business coach and dear friend, Luly Carerras, there are not words to thank you for how you impacted my life. You welcomed me, loved me, coached me, and believed in me in a time when fear was overwhelming and blinding. Meeting you was one of the greatest gifts of my life. Thank you for showing up as you and for being willing to be vulnerable and honest to guide me towards my path. Your compassion and empathy will forever be etched on my heart.

To my tribe, thank you for taking time to follow my work, watch my Facebook live videos, and spread my message with like-minded individuals. It is an honor to serve you and share my passion with you. I am extremely grateful for all my opportunities to support clients with massive breakthroughs. I genuinely love helping other people see their power. Helping others find their unique wellness brings me great joy. It is an amazing gift to see clients overcome their traumas and become the person of their dreams. It fills my heart over brim to hear stories of emotional transformation. Together, we can bring emotional and physical well-being to the world.

To my family, I thank you for allowing me to be myself. For enduring the hardships during my evolution and loving me through the process. I know the journey wasn't easy, but I do appreciate all of your support. My husband – he married a young, quiet, scared girl and lived through my evolution as I became an outspoken, confident, and passionate woman. My mom is my biggest fan – she always was and always will be. She watches every video, reads every post, and is sure to put in her two cents. I love her for her honesty, even if it's painful sometimes. My dad is my proudest fan – seeing him beam with pride over my accomplishments and enjoying our bonding time outdoors relaxing. My brother and sister, Carlos and Joanne, for being my guardians and supporters throughout my life. Thank you for understanding when I was distant and quiet during this process of evolution.

Finally, to my sons Gabriel and Lucas. Thank you for inspiring me and giving me the strength I needed to push through my illness and become the amazing mom you deserved. Thank you for your sense of humor, your gentleness, your love, your hugs, and your acceptance. You two are my everything and I live my life to honor you both. May my legacy make you proud.

ABOUT THE AUTHOR

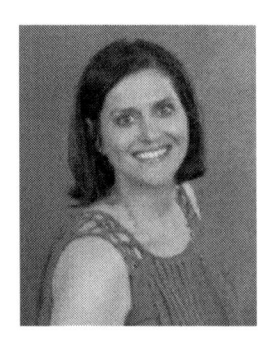

Diane Vich is a registered nurse, nursing professor, hypnotist and holistic health coach who helps people overcome chronic illness and pain through mind, body and soul connection. Through her own experience healing herself with alternative therapies, Diane helps clients overcome trauma, chronic disease and negative patterns that impact their health.

Diane's transformation began when she adopted holistic healing modalities while facing a debilitating illness, pain and fatigue that required her to take more than 13 prescription medications daily. Through nutrition, supplementation, climactic stretch, hypnosis and emotional healing, Diane not only transformed her health but reconnected with her long lost sexuality.

Diane now helps women connect with their sexual power and heal past trauma through workshops and coaching. She believes that sacred sexual energy is the key to creativity, power, self-actualization and fulfillment.

Diane currently lives in Miami, Florida, USA. And in her free time she enjoys the beach and outdoors with her husband and two children. She also loves supporting the community through education, counseling, children's books and innovation to transform the lives of children and families.

If you are sick and tired of anxiety, gut issues or chronic pain, and want to talk to someone that has felt your pain, schedule your Free Discovery call today. You have nothing to lose and everything to gain, you deserve to find your own unique wellness. Schedule your Free Discovery call today at https://calendly.com/dianevich/discovery

Website: http://dianevich.com
Social Links: linktr.ee/dianevich
Email: coachdianevich@gmail.com
Podcast:https://dreamvisions7radio.com/goddess-unleashed-diane-vich/
Facebook:https://www.facebook.com/dianevichgoddessunleashed/

Thank You

I want to thank you from the bottom of my heart for making the decision and taking the time to read *The Truth About IBS and Anxiety: Erasing the Symptoms Effortlessly*. If you have made it this far I know a few things about you already. First, you are vested in your own personal health journey and looking to improve your symptoms easily and effortlessly. And second, you were intrigued by my story and felt a connection with my pain. Or maybe, you are one of those people that check out the end of the book before you dive deep.

As a token of my appreciation and thanks for reaching out I would like to offer you a short class: *How to Thrive in Life with IBS and Anxiety*. It's a class with much more value than just insight on IBS and Anxiety. It's a course about overcoming chronic illness, chronic pain, autoimmune disease, carpel tunnel, pyriformis syndrome, EDS III, GERD, etc. It's a truly powerful tool to overcome the obstacles and challenges your Medical Diagnosis may be bringing into your life. Watch the free course at **https://dianevich.com/resources/**

I would love to learn more about your unique journey and success in overcoming your own unique illness, disease, trauma or pain. Please keep in touch and share your wins on Facebook or Instagram (tag me and use #IBScure #IBSandAnxietyguru #thrivewithIBS #thrivewithanxiety #selfcareisselflove or #goddessunleashed).

Feel Free to Follow me for more Tips, Hacks and Tricks to Thrive in Life:
linktr.ee/dianevich

Thank You Again for taking the time to read this book.

Printed in Great Britain
by Amazon